HUMAN SEXUALITY TO ACCOMPANY
Essential Health Skills

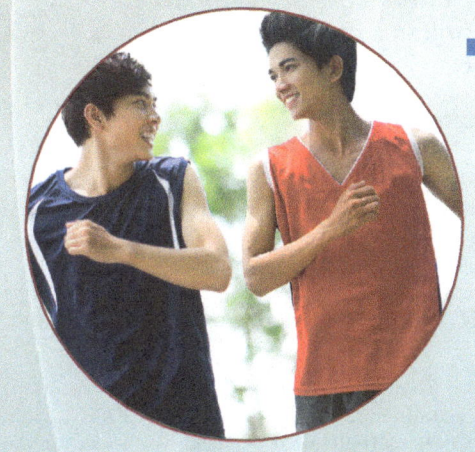

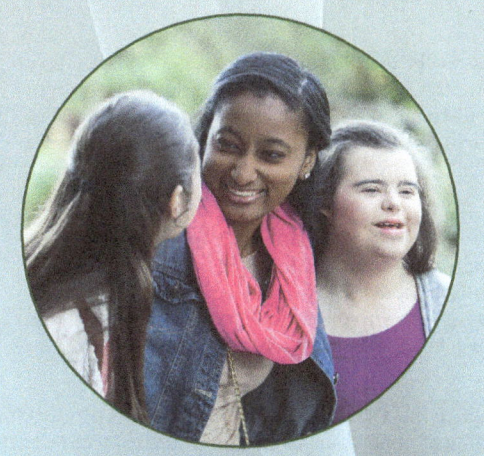

Catherine A. Sanderson, PhD
Professor of Psychology
Amherst College
Amherst, Massachusetts

Mark Zelman, PhD
Professor of Biology
Aurora University
Aurora, Illinois

Pedagogy Developers

Diane Farthing, NBCT
Health Educator
Pleasanton, California

Melanie Lynch, M.Ed.
Health Education Specialist
Pittsburgh, Pennsylvania

Melissa Munsell
Instructional Specialist
Physical Education and Health Department
San Antonio, Texas

Publisher
The Goodheart-Willcox Company, Inc.
Tinley Park, Illinois
www.g-w.com

Copyright © 2021
by
The Goodheart-Willcox Company, Inc.

All rights reserved. No part of this work may be reproduced, stored, or transmitted in any form or by any electronic or mechanical means, including information storage and retrieval systems, without the prior written permission of
The Goodheart-Willcox Company, Inc.

Manufactured in the United States of America.

ISBN 978-1-64564-433-0

4 5 6 7 8 9 — 21 — 25 24 23 22 21

The Goodheart-Willcox Company, Inc. Brand Disclaimer: Brand names, company names, and illustrations for products and services included in this text are provided for educational purposes only and do not represent or imply endorsement or recommendation by the author or the publisher.

The Goodheart-Willcox Company, Inc. CDC Disclaimer: The use of materials from the CDC (Centers for Disease Control and Prevention) used in Goodheart-Willcox textbooks and supplements does not imply endorsement or recommendation by the CDC, ATSDR (Agency for Toxic Substances and Disease Registry), HHS (Department of Health and Human Services), or the United States Government for the content, products, or services contained in Goodheart-Willcox print or digital publications. Materials from the CDC are also available at http://www.cdc.gov free of charge.

The Goodheart-Willcox Company, Inc. Safety Notice: The reader is expressly advised to carefully read, understand, and apply all safety precautions and warnings described in this book or that might also be indicated in undertaking the activities and exercises described herein to minimize risk of personal injury or injury to others. Common sense and good judgment should also be exercised and applied to help avoid all potential hazards. The reader should always refer to the appropriate manufacturer's technical information, directions, and recommendations; then proceed with care to follow specific equipment operating instructions. The reader should understand these notices and cautions are not exhaustive.

The publisher makes no warranty or representation whatsoever, either expressed or implied, including but not limited to equipment, procedures, and applications described or referred to herein, their quality, performance, merchantability, or fitness for a particular purpose. The publisher assumes no responsibility for any changes, errors, or omissions in this book. The publisher specifically disclaims any liability whatsoever, including any direct, indirect, incidental, consequential, special, or exemplary damages resulting, in whole or in part, from the reader's use or reliance upon the information, instructions, procedures, warnings, cautions, applications, or other matter contained in this book. The publisher assumes no responsibility for the activities of the reader.

The Goodheart-Willcox Company, Inc. Internet Disclaimer: The Internet resources and listings in this Goodheart-Willcox Publisher product are provided solely as a convenience to you. These resources and listings were reviewed at the time of publication to provide you with accurate, safe, and appropriate information. Goodheart-Willcox Publisher has no control over the referenced websites and, due to the dynamic nature of the Internet, is not responsible or liable for the content, products, or performance of links to other websites or resources. Goodheart-Willcox Publisher makes no representation, either expressed or implied, regarding the content of these websites, and such references do not constitute an endorsement or recommendation of the information or content presented. It is your responsibility to take all protective measures to guard against inappropriate content, viruses, or other destructive elements.

Cover images: Left column, top to bottom: Dragon Images/Shutterstock.com, kali9/E+/GettyImages, Tirachard/iStock/Getty Images Plus/GettyImages; Right image: Dmytro Zinkevych/Shutterstock.com
Blue background element: ArtFish/Shutterstock.com
Big Ideas icon: Hilch/Shutterstock.com
Health Management Plan icon: IconBunny/Shutterstock.com
Skills icon: Goodheart-Willcox Publisher
Reading and Notetaking icon: Webicon/Shutterstock.com
Setting the Scene icon: Legend_art/Shutterstock.com
Research in Action icon: Lucky Creative/Shutterstock.com
Health in the Media icon: Dacian G/Shutterstock.com
Case Study icon: FishCoolish/Shutterstock.com
Quiz icon: VectorKnight/Shutterstock.com
Local and Global Health icon: Oleh Svetiukha/Shutterstock.com
Spotlight on Health and Wellness Careers icon: Imagine Room/Shutterstock.com
Health Across the Life Span background: Triff/Shutterstock.com

About the Authors

Catherine A. Sanderson is the Manwell Family Professor of Life Sciences (Psychology) at Amherst College. She received a bachelor's degree in psychology, with a specialization in Health and Development, from Stanford University, and received both master's and doctoral degrees in psychology from Princeton University. Professor Sanderson's research examines how personality and social variables influence health-related behaviors, such as safer sex and disordered eating. Her research also examines the development of persuasive messages and interventions to prevent unhealthy behavior and predictors of relationship satisfaction. This research has received grant funding from the National Science Foundation and the National Institutes of Health. Professor Sanderson has published more than 25 journal articles and book chapters; four college textbooks; high school and middle school health textbooks; and a trade book, *The Positive Shift*, which examines how mind-set influences happiness, health, and even how long people live. Her latest book, *Why We Act: Turning Bystanders into Moral Rebels*, examines why good people often stay silent or do nothing in the face of wrongdoing. In 2012, she was named one of the country's top 300 professors by the Princeton Review.

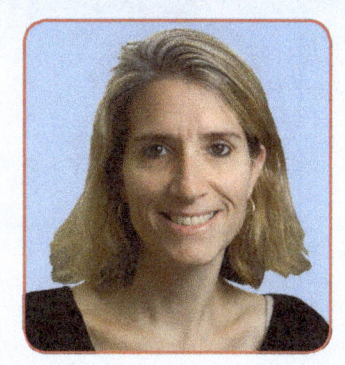

Mark Zelman is a Professor of Biology at Aurora University, Aurora, Illinois. He received a bachelor's degree in biology at Rockford College, with minors in chemistry and psychology. He received a PhD in microbiology and immunology at Loyola University of Chicago, where he studied the molecular and cellular mechanisms of autoimmune disease. During his postdoctoral research at the University of Chicago, he studied aspects of cell physiology pertaining to cell growth and cancer. Dr. Zelman supervises undergraduate research on streptococcal and staphylococcal infections, and mechanisms of antibiotic resistance. He teaches science education courses for high school teachers. He has published articles on microbiology, infectious disease, autoimmune disease, and biotechnology, and he has written two college texts on human diseases and infection control. Dr. Zelman works with the West Africa AIDS Foundation and other public health projects in the US and abroad. He is an officer of the Illinois State Academy of Sciences.

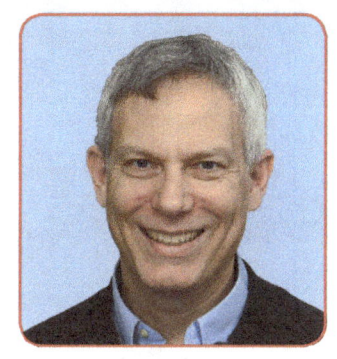

Pedagogy Developers

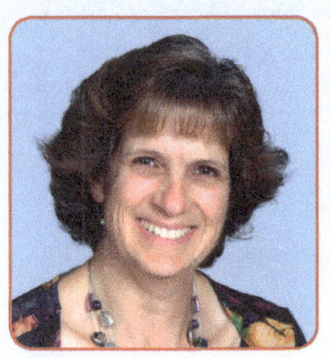

Diane Farthing received her bachelor's degree and teaching credentials from Kent State University in Ohio and has been teaching health education for 37 years. In 2010, she became a National Board Certified Teacher. Diane's teaching career includes 16 years at a continuation high school and five years at the middle school level. Since 2004, she has been teaching health education and anatomy and physiology at Amador Valley High School in Pleasanton. She is a strong believer in the power of collaboration. She spent seven years as part of the Bay Area Physical Education-Health Subject Matter Project leadership team designing and delivering professional development institutes. In 2014, she took on the role of Health Program Director for the Health and Physical Education Collaborative (H-PEC), a nonprofit organization dedicated to helping teachers develop physical and health literacy in their students. Diane was a member of the CDE's Framework and Evaluation Criteria Committee and helped write the Health Education Curriculum Framework for California Public Schools. She is the 2019 California Association for Health, Physical Education, Recreation, and Dance (CAHPERD) Health Teacher of the Year and the 2020 Western District Teacher of the Year.

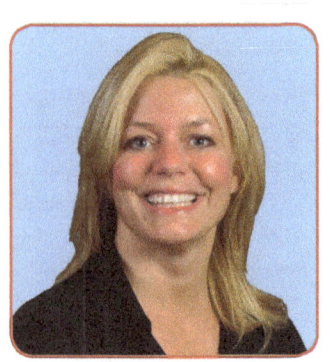

Melanie Lynch is an experienced teacher with more than 25 years in the classroom. She spent the first 21 years of her career specializing in teaching only health education. She now teaches health and physical education in Pittsburgh, Pennsylvania, at North Allegheny Intermediate High School. She has served as Vice President of Health Education for SHAPE Pennsylvania for five years and served as their President in 2016. Also in 2016, SHAPE America named Melanie the National Health Education Teacher of the Year. Melanie's love of working with students and her creative, skills-based lesson ideas have taken her all over the country, where she has spoken to thousands of teachers. Melanie is grateful to work, learn, and grow with so many amazing teachers.

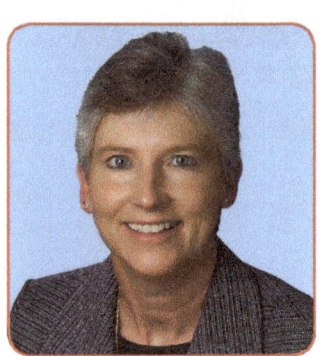

Melissa Munsell has worked as an instructional specialist in the Physical Education and Health Department at North East Independent School District in San Antonio, Texas, and served as the K–12 Health Education Lead for the district. Melissa received a bachelor's degree in kinesiology from The University of Texas at Austin and is certified to teach Physical Education K–12 and Health Education 6–12, among other endorsements, in the state of Texas. She has 26 years of teaching and administrative experience, including six years teaching health education at the high school level. She has also served as vice president of the Health Division and General Division of the Texas Association for Health, Physical Education, Recreation, and Dance (TAHPERD) and presents workshops and lectures on various health topics locally and statewide.

Contributors and Reviewers

Contributors

Goodheart-Willcox Publisher would like to thank the following classroom instructor who contributed to the development of the *Warm-Up*, *Real World Health Skills*, *Health and Wellness Skills*, and *Hands-On Activities*.

Haillie Moudy
Health and Physical Education Instructor
Sierra Sands Unified School District
Ridgecrest, California

Advisory Board

Goodheart-Willcox Publisher would like to thank the following advisory board members who provided guidance in the development of *Human Sexuality*.

Carolyn Cleaves
Health Instructor
Alisal High School
Salinas, California

Susan Gabin
Health Educator
Frontier High School
Bakersfield, California

Mary Irilian
Health Instructor
Hart High School
Newhall, California

Kellie A. Johnson
Assistant Athletic Coordinator, Health Instructor
LEE High School
San Antonio, Texas

Beth Kahn
Health Instructor
North Salinas High School
Salinas, California

Janelle Merry
Health and Physical Education Instructor
North County Trade Technical High School
Vista, California

Haillie Moudy
Health and Physical Education Instructor
Sierra Sands Unified School District
Ridgecrest, California

Tracey Rudnick
Health Instructor
Bradley Middle School
San Antonio, Texas

Nancy Searle
Health Instructor
McCallum High School
Austin, Texas

Shasta Smith
Health Education Instructor
Sitka High School
Sitka, Alaska

Delia Thibodeaux
Health Instructor
Westside High School
Houston, Texas

Goodheart-Willcox Publisher would also like to thank the members of the **2019 CAHPERD Convention Focus Group**, who shared feedback and insight that influenced the development of this book.

Instructor Reviewers

Goodheart-Willcox Publisher would like to thank the following health education instructors who reviewed selected chapters and contributed valuable input into the development of *Human Sexuality*.

Kyle Bell
Health/Physical Education Instructor
Canyon High School
Anaheim Hills, California

Haillie Moudy
Health and Physical Education Instructor
Sierra Sands Unified School District
Ridgecrest, California

Heather R. Perrigan
Professional Health Educator
Corvallis High School
Corvallis, Oregon

Mary Record
High School Health Instructor
Scarborough High School
Scarborough, Maine

Dr. Chuck Rhoades
Health Instructor
Portsmouth High School
Portsmouth, New Hampshire

Cynthia Smyser
Science and Health Instructor
University of Illinois Laboratory
   High School
Urbana, Illinois

James Tulley
Health Education Instructor
Scarsdale High School
Scarsdale, New York

Contents

Chapter 23 **Understanding Sexuality** **800**

    Lesson 23.1 Aspects of Sexuality 802

    Lesson 23.2 Sexual Feelings and Behavior 811

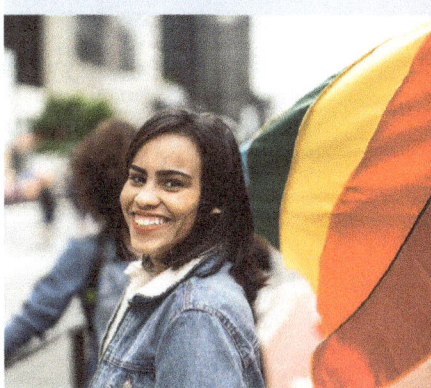

Chapter 24 **Pregnancy Prevention** **824**

    Lesson 24.1 What Is Contraception? 826

    Lesson 24.2 Barrier Methods 833

    Lesson 24.3 Hormonal Methods 839

    Lesson 24.4 Natural Methods and Sterilization 846

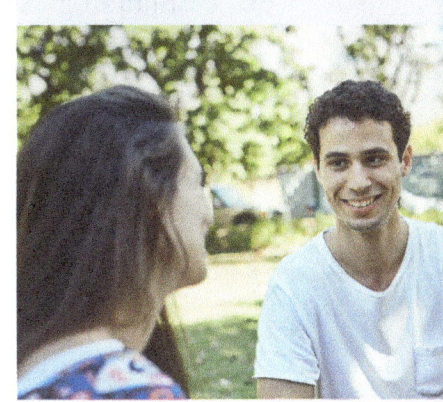

Glossary/Glosario 856

Index 860

Feature Contents

Case Studies

The LGBT+ Community 808
Is That Really True? 829

Research in Action

Children of Same-Sex Parents 809
Hormonal Contraceptives for Males 844

Local and Global Health

The Evolving View of Biological Sex 804
The Impact of the Pill 841

Health in the Media

Portrayal of Sex in the Media 816
Media Messages About Contraception 827

Skills for Health and Wellness

Use the Decision-Making Process: Sexual Activity 817
Answering Questions About Your Sexual Health 831

To the Student

We wrote an exciting textbook, *Essential Health Skills*, for high school health and wellness classes based on our experiences as professors of psychology (Catherine Sanderson) and biology (Mark Zelman), and as the accomplished authors of high school and college-level textbooks.

As a supplement to the textbook, we created *Human Sexuality* to align with the National Sexuality Education Standards. Picking up where the textbook leaves off, *Human Sexuality* covers topics from gender identity to sexual decision-making and pregnancy prevention. As with our textbook, we wanted this supplement to give high school students the most current sexual health information, presented in an engaging writing style so students would enjoy reading the book. Additionally, we included a focus on practical health skills that young people can use to develop and promote positive health and wellness habits throughout their lives.

As the authors of high school and college-level textbooks, we felt confident in our research and writing abilities, but felt that the pedagogy was better left to health teachers. We would like to thank Diane Farthing, Melanie Lynch, and Melissa Munsell for developing the skills-based questions, activities, and resources that are a vital part of this course. We are delighted with the final product, and wish all readers of this book a lifetime of health.

Chapter 23: Understanding Sexuality

Lesson 23.1 Aspects of Sexuality
Lesson 23.2 Sexual Feelings and Behavior

Look for the skills icon throughout this chapter for opportunities to practice your health skills.

Check Your Health and Wellness Skills

In this chapter, you will learn skills for making healthy decisions about sexuality. To understand the skills you currently use, take the following inventory of your behaviors. Indicate how well you think you use each skill. Use a scale of 1–5, *1* meaning you do not use the skill and *5* meaning you feel completely comfortable using it.

Skill	How Well Do You Use Each Skill?
I understand that sexuality is a normal part of development.	
I show respect for people of different sexes, gender identities, and sexual orientations.	
I feel confident in who I am, whether I fit gender stereotypes or not.	
I speak up if I witness other people showing homophobia.	
I know that portrayals of sex in the media aren't usually realistic.	
I understand my own values and beliefs about sexual activity.	
I know how the consequences of a sexual relationship could change my future.	
I discuss my expectations, consent, and boundaries about sexual activity with a partner.	
I respect others' consent and boundaries about sexual activity.	
I use the decision-making process to make healthy decisions about sexual activity.	
	Total:

Add up your responses to each statement. The higher your score, the more comfortable you feel making healthy decisions about sexuality. Which skill do you think is most important for you? Which skill is the most challenging for you? Which skill would you most like to improve? In this chapter, you will learn how to perform these skills better and more often.

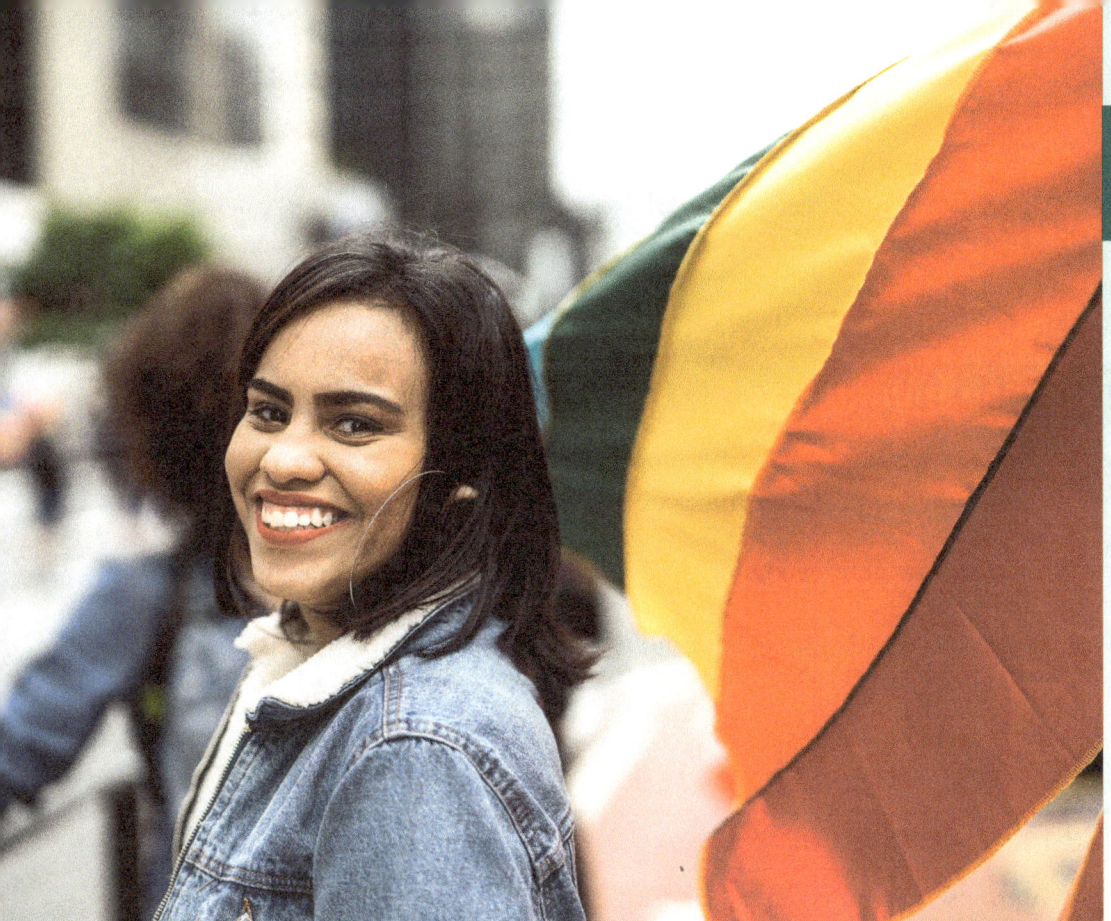

FG Trade/E+/Getty Images

Reading and Notetaking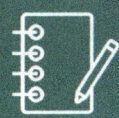

Before you hear about the content in this chapter, think about how you would answer the following questions:
- What is sexuality?
- Are sexual orientation and gender identity the same thing?
- What are the consequences of sexual relationships?

As you listen to your teacher present this lesson, take notes about these topics using a graphic organizer like the one shown. Use the text to add any additional notes you may have missed.

What is sexuality?	
Are sexual orientation and gender identity the same thing?	
What are the consequences of sexual relationships?	

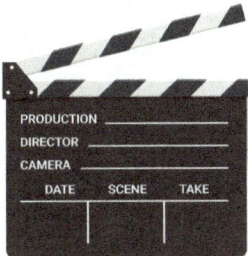

Setting the Scene

Views of Sexuality

After you attended a very small middle school, life at your new high school is full of exciting opportunities and challenges. One of these challenges is adjusting to the culture at your new school. In your middle school, most students had similar views about sexuality. At your new high school, people have many different attitudes about sex, sexuality, and how people of the same or opposite sex should interact.

You know you are not the only one going through this adjustment. Some of your classmates from middle school make fun of students who have different views. You know this approach is wrong, however. You do not have to compromise your own values and decisions to respect others. You want to learn more about the different attitudes of your classmates, but sometimes it feels awkward or scary to ask.

Thinking Critically

1. What factors have influenced your views on sex and sexuality?
2. How are your views on sex and sexuality different from the views of your peers? How are your views similar?
3. Why is it important to respect other people's views about sex and sexuality? What questions could you ask to learn more about a person's views?

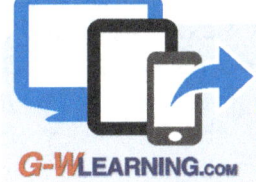

Click on the activity icon or visit www.g-wlearning.com/health/4330 to access online vocabulary activities using key terms from the chapter.

Lesson 23.1 Aspects of Sexuality

Essential Question?
What qualities and behaviors make up a person's sexuality?

Key Terms

cisgender
disorder of sex development (DSD)
gender binary
gender identity
gender nonconforming
homophobia
LGBT+
nonbinary
same-sex marriage
sexuality
sexual orientation
transgender

Learning Outcomes

After studying this lesson, you will be able to
- identify the aspects that make up a person's sexuality;
- explain how biological sex is assigned;
- describe how gender identity and expression influence a person's sexuality;
- analyze different sexual and romantic orientations; and
- assess the importance of support for individuals who are LGBT+.

✓ Warm-Up Activity

Gender Stereotypes

Comprehend Concepts
Gender stereotypes are assumptions made about an individual based on gender. Before reading this lesson, think of a trait commonly associated with a gender stereotype you have encountered. For example, your trait might be "being good at math" or "being sensitive." Take turns reading each trait to the class. If you relate to the trait described in a statement, stand up. Once all statements have been read, discuss observations as a class. Did the pattern of who stood up or stayed seated fit feminine or masculine stereotypes? Why or why not? Then, discuss how gender stereotypes can be harmful.

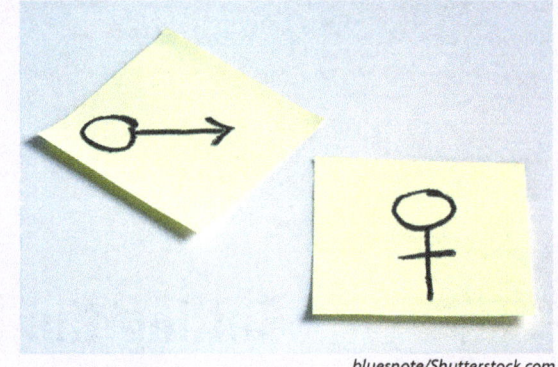

bluesnote/Shutterstock.com

sexuality element of identity that includes a person's biological sex, gender identity and expression, sexual orientation, and sexual experiences and thoughts

When you hear the word *sexuality*, what do you think of? Maybe you think about your decision to abstain from sexual activity or your sexual orientation. Sexuality includes these factors, but it also includes other aspects of your identity. You do not have to be sexually active to explore and understand your sexuality.

Sexuality is an important part of identity and is the expression of gender and sexual feelings. It includes how you look, feel, think, and behave (**Figure 23.1**). It also affects how other people perceive and treat you and the roles you play in your family and in society.

Biological Sex

Biological sex refers to whether you are genetically and physically male or female. The sex chromosomes you inherited from your biological parents determine your biological sex. Eggs and sperm contain these sex chromosomes. If both the egg and the sperm contribute X chromosomes, a person will be female. If the sperm contributes a Y chromosome, a person will have one X chromosome and one Y chromosome and be male. Sex chromosomes direct the development and growth of the reproductive organs and other sexual characteristics. Much of this growth and development occurred before you were born.

How Biological Sex Is Assigned

Though biological sex is usually assigned at birth, doctors can often detect a person's biological sex even before birth. At about the seventh week of prenatal development, a doctor can use a blood test to determine a baby's biological sex. After the 18th week of development, an ultrasound can help visualize a baby's reproductive organs. Typically, a doctor can determine a baby's biological sex at birth by observing the external reproductive organs. According to this observation, the baby is assigned a biological sex. For this reason, biological sex is sometimes called *assigned sex*.

Disorders of Sex Development (DSDs)

Most babies can be identified at birth as either male or female. Some babies, however, are born with or develop an ambiguous, or unclear, biological sex. This condition is called a **disorder of sex development (DSD)**, though some people prefer to call it a *difference of sex development (DSD)* or *intersex*. DSDs are relatively common, occurring in as many as 1–2 percent of live births. Babies with DSDs have external reproductive organs that are not obviously male or female.

In most cases, DSDs occur because reproductive organs have not developed fully and cannot be identified. For example, male organs may appear small or resemble female organs. In other cases, external reproductive organs do not match a baby's chromosomal sex. That is, some babies with XY chromosomes are born with female characteristics, and some babies with XX chromosomes develop male characteristics. When this occurs, doctors may order blood tests to identify the baby's sex chromosomes and the type of DSD. These tests and the baby's anatomy help parents understand the baby's sexual development. Parents may assign a sex to the baby and choose to raise the baby as male or female. These babies may or may not grow up comfortable with their assigned sex.

Some sex chromosome combinations cause ambiguous sexual development later in life. For example, babies with *Turner Syndrome* have one X chromosome from one parent and no sex chromosome from the other. *Klinefelter Syndrome* describes the presence of two X chromosomes and one Y chromosome. Babies with Turner Syndrome or Klinefelter Syndrome do not show signs of ambiguity at birth. Instead, their sexually ambiguous traits appear during puberty. These observations indicate that being male or female is more complicated than possessing certain sexual anatomy or sex chromosomes.

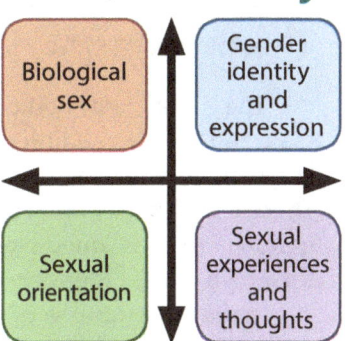

Figure 23.1 Your sexuality involves more than just your sexual orientation or sexual behaviors.

disorder of sex development (DSD) condition of being born with or developing an ambiguous biological sex; also called a *difference of sex development (DSD)* or *intersex*

Local and Global Health

The Evolving View of Biological Sex

The United States officially recognizes two sexes: male and female. Medical professionals have long known that a small percentage of children have DSDs. These children may face challenges as they grow and mature if their assigned biological sex conflicts with their own gender identity.

In the US, a number of states are adapting to science's improved understanding of gender and sex. For example, some states allow people to identify as *male*, *female*, or *X* on their driver's licenses. This is more inclusive of people who are nonbinary. Many US businesses and other organizations also give people the option to select a third sex for documents such as airline tickets and college applications.

This evolving view of gender and sex is also evident around the world. In 2013, Germany became the first European country to allow parents to assign a third sex to a child born with an ambiguous biological sex. Norway recognizes that adults may want to change their assigned sex. Adults in Norway can do this by submitting paperwork to the government and do not need a doctor's recommendation or surgery. Australia recently enacted a law to protect people with DSDs from discrimination.

Practice Your Skills

Advocate for Health

People who have DSDs may or may not be comfortable with the biological sex they are assigned at birth. With a partner, search online or read an article or book about a person with a DSD. Read about this person's experience, feelings, and challenges. Then, with your partner, discuss what steps you could take to increase awareness and acceptance for people with DSDs in your community. What small changes could your community make to help people with DSDs feel more accepted? What information do you think people in your community need to know about DSDs? Then, create a communication campaign to spread these messages in your community. Adapt the information for your audience and share this information on social media, through flyers, or in a public service announcement (PSA).

Gender

Gender describes the characteristics a society associates with a biological sex. These expectations vary among societies and cultures and change over time. For example, some people believe in strict *gender roles*, or behaviors considered "appropriate" for each gender. Some people also have *gender stereotypes*, or assumptions based on gender. These traits, roles, and stereotypes influence how people think and behave.

The Gender Binary

Movies, advertisements, and other media often present unrealistic, exaggerated images of the traits associated with *masculinity* (being male) and *femininity* (being female). In some cases, the media implies that extreme masculinity and femininity are normal and desirable. These influences, along with other cultural and societal influences, can lead to extremely opposite perceptions of what it means to be male or female (**Figure 23.2**).

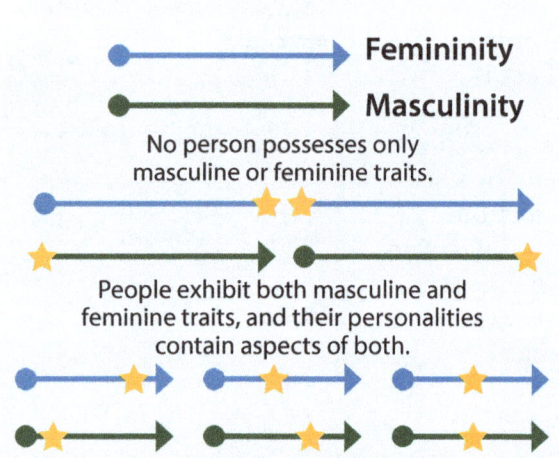

Figure 23.2 Most people's behavior lies somewhere between the extremes of completely feminine and completely masculine. *What is the name of the idea that the genders of man and woman are opposites?*

These perceptions are an example of the **gender binary**, or the idea that the genders of man and woman are entirely opposite. Seeing gender this way is unrealistic. No person exhibits traits associated with each gender to the extreme, and no one can attain them to the degree portrayed by the media.

For these reasons, the expression of masculinity and femininity can be a source of insecurity. People may feel insecure about the way others perceive them. They think they are supposed to be entirely "masculine" or "feminine," not realizing these are just descriptions, or stereotypes, and not something that exists in real individuals.

gender binary view that the genders of man and woman are entirely opposite; ignores gender expressions that fall between these opposites

gender identity component of identity that describes deeply held thoughts and feelings about one's gender

Gender Identity and Expression

Gender identity describes a person's internal, deeply held thoughts and feelings about gender. Gender identity influences a person's *gender expression*, or outward display of gender. Gender expression includes the way a person dresses, acts, and talks. It also includes how a person wants to be treated by others (**Figure 23.3**).

A child's sense of gender becomes well-established around five years of age. During childhood, most boys will play with other boys, and girls will play with other girls. This may be a way for children to solidify and support their own sense of gender identity. It is normal, however, for some children to role-play as the opposite sex or prefer to play with children of the opposite sex.

Gender Identities

Gender Identity	Description
Agender	Having a gender identity that does not align with woman, man, or any other gender; also called *gender neutral*
Androgynous	Exhibiting masculine and feminine traits equally
Bigender	Having a gender identity that includes both man and woman
Cisgender	Having a gender identity that matches one's biological sex assigned at birth
Gender fluid	Having a changing, or *fluid*, gender identity
Gender nonconforming	Having a gender identity that does not follow gender expectations based on a person's biological sex assigned at birth
Gender questioning	Being unsure about one's gender identity or experimenting with different genders
Nonbinary	Having a gender identity that falls outside or between the categories of man and woman; also called *gender queer*
Transgender	Having a gender identity that does not match one's biological sex assigned at birth

Figure 23.3 Each term describes how a person may identify with gender.

Most people identify with the gender associated with their biological sex. These people are called **cisgender**. Some people realize they are not comfortable with the gender associated with their biological sex. This happens for many reasons. People who identify with a gender that does not match their biological sex are called **gender nonconforming**.

For example, a person with female reproductive organs may be raised as a girl, but later in life feel like a boy, regardless of anatomy or chromosomes. This person may choose to identify as a man and assume the associated role and behaviors. This person is considered to be **transgender**. People who are transgender identify with the gender opposite their biological sex. A woman who is transgender is born with male sexual anatomy, but identifies as a woman. A man who is transgender is born with female sexual anatomy, but identifies as a man. Some people who are transgender choose to change their appearance, clothing, and name to match the gender with which they identify.

Other people who are gender nonconforming may be **nonbinary**. This means they have a gender identity that falls outside the categories of man or woman. These people may identify with neither gender (*agender*) or both genders (*bigender*). Some people may have a *fluid*, or changing, gender identity.

cisgender identifying with the gender associated with one's biological sex

gender nonconforming identifying with a gender that is not associated with one's biological sex

transgender identifying with the gender opposite the one that is associated with one's biological sex

nonbinary identifying with a gender that falls outside the categories of man or woman

Sexual Orientation

sexual orientation
enduring pattern of a person's romantic and/or sexual attraction to other people

A person's sexual orientation is separate from gender identity. People of all gender identities can have any orientation. **Sexual orientation** describes the enduring pattern of a person's romantic and/or sexual attraction to other people. *Sexual attraction* involves interest in a person's physical qualities and desire for sexual activity with that person. *Romantic attraction* is a feeling of emotional connection to another person and the desire for an intimate relationship. Some people use the word *romantic orientation* to describe a person's romantic attraction. People of various orientations are not necessarily attracted or unattracted to all people of a particular gender. Differences in personality, appearance, and gender expression all play a role in how attractive someone finds a person.

Sexual and romantic orientation correlate for many, but not all, people. For example, even though people who are asexual do not experience sexual attraction, some do experience romantic attraction. **Figure 23.4** contains some of the terms used to describe sexual and romantic orientation.

Sexual and Romantic Orientations

Sexual Orientations

Sexual Orientation	Description
Heterosexual	Having sexual attraction for people of the opposite gender; also called *straight*
Homosexual	Having sexual attraction for people of the same gender; sometimes called *gay* or *lesbian*
Androsexual	Having sexual attraction for masculinity
Gynesexual	Having sexual attraction for femininity
Bisexual	Having sexual attraction for both men and women
Polysexual	Having sexual attraction for multiple genders (including nonbinary genders)
Skoliosexual	Having sexual attraction for people who are nonbinary
Pansexual	Having sexual attraction for all genders (including nonbinary genders)
Demisexual	Developing sexual attraction only with a deep emotional bond
Asexual	Not having any sexual attraction for other people

Romantic Orientations

Romantic Orientation	Description
Heteroromantic	Having romantic attraction for people of the opposite gender
Homoromantic	Having romantic attraction for people of the same gender
Androromantic	Having romantic attraction for masculinity
Gyneromantic	Having romantic attraction for femininity
Biromantic	Having romantic attraction for both men and women
Polyromantic	Having romantic attraction for multiple genders (including nonbinary genders)
Skolioromantic	Having romantic attraction for people who are nonbinary
Panromantic	Having romantic attraction for all genders (including nonbinary genders)
Demiromantic	Developing romantic attraction only with a deep emotional bond
Aromantic	Not having any romantic attraction for other people

Figure 23.4 Everyone has both a sexual orientation and a romantic orientation. *Can a person's romantic orientation be different from sexual orientation? Give an example.*

People of all orientations can be found in all races, ethnicities, cultures, countries, and social and economic backgrounds. People who are unsure about their orientation are often called *questioning*. Many factors, some unknown, influence the development of a person's sexual orientation. Known factors include a person's genes, environment, and experiences.

It is not unusual for some teens to be unsure of or confused about their sexual orientation. At times, some teens who are heterosexual feel romantic or sexual attraction to people of the same gender. This does not necessarily mean they are nonheterosexual. For example, a girl might develop a "crush" on another girl in her school or on a female celebrity. This type of sexual curiosity is fairly common while adolescents are maturing and is due in part to increased hormone levels. In time, most teens sort out their feelings and understand their sexual orientation (**Figure 23.5**).

Support for LGBT+ Youth

During adolescence, teens are exploring their sexuality. Regardless of their gender identity and sexual orientation, teens think about and want to discuss their feelings and dating experiences. Teens who are gender nonconforming, nonbinary, and nonheterosexual often feel, however, that they must hide this part of themselves from others. Hiding this part of identity is sometimes called being *closeted* or *in the closet*.

LGBT+ is a common acronym used to identify people of these sexual orientations and gender identities. It stands for *lesbian*, *gay*, *bisexual*, and *transgender*. The plus sign indicates the inclusion of other sexual orientations and gender identities as well. For example, the acronym *LGBT* is sometimes expanded to include *Q* (queer or questioning), *I* (intersex), and *A* (asexual). Some people argue that, despite efforts to be inclusive, this acronym does not represent every sexual orientation or gender identity. Additionally, not everyone wants to be defined by this acronym. As the LGBT+ community evolves, so will the terminology used to describe it.

LGBT+ acronym used to identify people who are nonheterosexual and/or gender nonconforming

LGBT+ Discrimination

Generally, people who are LGBT+ are accepted more widely today than in the past. Still, these individuals experience varying degrees of prejudice, rejection, bullying, sexual harassment, and violence.

Questions About Sexual Orientation

Do not put pressure on yourself. Many people need time to explore their identities throughout their teen years, and even during their whole lives.
You do not have to decide on one label, and even if you do, this may change in later years.

Ask yourself some questions and reflect honestly about how you feel. If you feel confused or upset about your gender identity or sexual orientation, trusted adults and professionals can listen and help.

Remember that dreams or fantasies may not indicate anything about your sexual orientation. They can, however, help you explore your feelings safely and privately without acting on them.

Figure 23.5 Throughout your teen years, you may find yourself developing sexual feelings toward a particular gender or biological sex. As you do, reflecting on these feelings can help you explore this aspect of your identity.

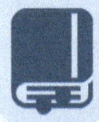

Case Study

The LGBT+ Community

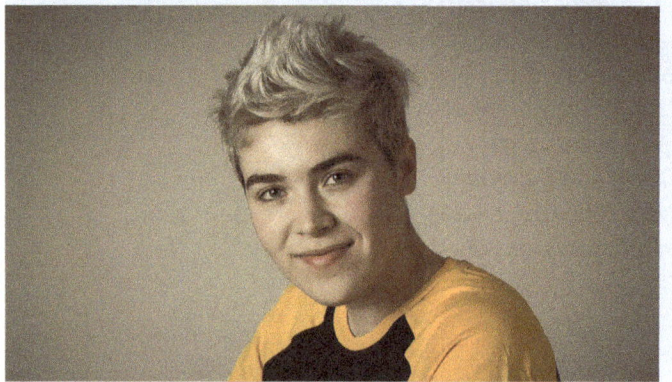

sam thomas/iStock / Getty Images Plus/Getty Images

Bailey took a big risk coming out to family members as gender nonbinary. Bailey's family had not talked much about LGBT+ people, so Bailey was not sure what to expect. Bailey was relieved when the family expressed support and understanding. Bailey's family members do occasionally forget to use Bailey's they/them pronouns, but Bailey can tell they are trying. A gentle reminder is all it takes for Bailey's family to remember the correct way to address them.

Growing up, Leesa was confused by her sexual orientation. When all her friends started to have crushes on boys or male celebrities, Leesa did not. She did not have crushes on girls either. For a while, Leesa feared something was wrong with her. When she read an article from an LGBT+ website about asexuality, she felt relieved and no longer felt alone. She recently joined a group on social media for people who are asexual and has made a few friends who share her experiences.

Dominick was walking out of school with his friend when he noticed Leah, a girl from his history class, being taunted by two other classmates. The two classmates were calling Leah degrading names, mocking her for being a lesbian, and blocking her path as she tried to walk away. Dominick turned to his friend and told him to find a teacher, while Dominick stepped in front of Leah. He told the two classmates to walk away and asked Leah if she was all right.

Practice Your Skills

Communicate with Others

Conversations about sexuality can be difficult to navigate, but are important to maintaining personal health and healthy relationships. In small groups, create a script scenario in which Bailey, Leesa, Dominick, or Leah has a conversation about sexuality. This conversation can be with a family member, friend, or trusted adult. Write the script using effective communication skills. Turn in your script to your teacher to share with the class.

Compared with their peers, teens who are LGBT+ have a greater risk of developing depression or anxiety, dropping out of school, running away from home, or attempting suicide. To avoid harassment, many people who are LGBT+ hide their sexual orientation or gender identity, although it can be difficult and painful to deny this basic part of who they are.

The term **homophobia** was first used in 1969 to describe an irrational fear of homosexuality. Today, it refers to hostility, anger, exclusion, and violence directed at people who are LGBT+. Teens who are LGBT+ may face the negative attitudes and actions associated with homophobia occasionally or on a daily basis.

Despite the discrimination that is still present, many teens who are LGBT+, especially those who have strong support systems, do feel comfortable with themselves. Many go through the process of "coming out" and tell trusted family members, friends, and others about their sexual orientation or gender identity. It is important for teens who are LGBT+ to have a supportive and accepting group of people around them. Many schools have student organizations for students who are LGBT+ and their *allies*, or students who support them. An example is a *gay straight alliance* or *GSA*.

homophobia hostility, anger, exclusion, and violence directed at people who are LGBT+

Laws Protecting LGBT+ Individuals

Governments have passed laws to protect people who are LGBT+ from discrimination. Federal laws, including the Civil Service Reform Act of 1978 and the Civil Rights Act of 1991, prohibit workplace discrimination against employees because of their sexual orientation or gender identity.

You read briefly about hate crimes in Chapter 15. *Hate crimes* are criminal acts motivated by the offender's bias against a person's actual or perceived race, religion, disability, ethnicity, gender identity, or sexual orientation. People who are LGBT+ are frequent targets of these crimes.

The Matthew Shepard and James Byrd, Jr., Hate Crimes Prevention Act protects people from crimes that target people because of their sexual orientation, gender identity, disability, and race. Matthew Shepard was a young man who was murdered because he was gay. James Byrd, Jr., was killed by a white supremacist because he was African-American.

On June 26, 2015, the US Supreme Court legalized **same-sex marriage**, or the legal marriage between two people of the same sex. This established that same-sex couples have the right to marry. Therefore, all states must issue marriage licenses to same-sex couples, and states must recognize same-sex marriages legally performed in other states. The court's decision was based on the Fourteenth Amendment of the US Constitution, which guarantees all US citizens have the same rights.

same-sex marriage legal marriage between two people of the same biological sex

Research in Action

Children of Same-Sex Parents

The US Census Bureau estimates about 105,000 children live in families with same-sex parents. Today, many of these same-sex parents are legally married.

The American Academy of Pediatrics (AAP), the leading organization for the scientific study of children's health in the US, reviewed more than 30 years of research about the well-being of children who have same-sex parents. The AAP concluded that having same-sex parents had no effect on children's emotional or physical health. Also, children fared as well having two male parents as they did having two female parents.

A recent study confirmed that family stability is the most important factor affecting children's health. This study found that the well-being of children was better if children's parents were legally married. This applied whether children had same-sex or opposite-sex parents.

 Practice Your Skills

Advocate for Health

Conduct research on new findings about same-sex parents. What new scientific evidence expands on the health effects of being raised by same-sex parents? Summarize your findings in small groups and explain why your resources are valid and reliable sources of health information.

In these same groups, assess how well your school promotes acceptance and tolerance among people of all sexual orientations and gender identities. Do people of all sexual orientations and gender identities feel accepted at your school? Are all family structures treated with respect? Examine what your school community does well and what it could do better. Together, brainstorm strategies your school community can use to foster an environment that promotes respect for other people.

Select a specific target audience for your information and choose the most effective method of communicating these strategies. Incorporate information from your research and provide resources for people who want more information.

Safe Zones

As teens who are LGBT+ learn more about their gender identity and sexual orientation, they may feel out of place and need support. Programs called *safe zones* are designed to help people in the LGBT+ community feel welcome. These programs are important for students who are LGBT+, since they are more likely to experience bullying and exclusion. High schools with these programs designate specific parts of the school as spaces where people will be accepted for who they are. This space could be a room, a particular staff member or teacher, or an entire school. A specific logo or symbol identifies this space. In a safe zone, students know they will be accepted and can discuss LGBT+ issues openly.

Providing safe zones increases inclusiveness and support in a school. One study conducted in a high school found that safe zones led to greater feelings of safety, tolerance, and respect for students who are LGBT+. Even subtle reminders of safe zones can lead to more positive feelings about school climate. Another study, conducted at the State University of New York, compared how students felt after seeing a syllabus that did or did not include a safe zone symbol. Students who saw the safe zone symbol said their college campus had a more positive climate for students who are LGBT+. These findings suggest that safe zone programs lead to an overall more positive school climate.

Lesson 23.1 Review

Know and Understand
1. Why is biological sex sometimes called *assigned sex*?
2. Why is the gender binary an unrealistic view?
3. Explain the difference between being cisgender, gender nonconforming, and nonbinary.
4. How is romantic attraction different from sexual attraction?
5. Give an example of what homophobia looks like today.

Think Critically
6. What factors do you think influence whether a person with a DSD grows up comfortable with the sex assigned at birth?
7. What are some examples of traits associated with the genders man and woman? How realistic are these traits, and how would believing them influence a person's health and decisions?
8. Why do you think people who are LGBT+ sometimes face discrimination? What steps can people take to help them feel welcome and accepted?

✓ REAL WORLD Health Skills

Practice Health-Enhancing Behaviors Individually or in small groups, brainstorm the different factors that you have observed influence gender stereotypes. Together, identify some ways teens at your school could combat or challenge these factors and change these stereotypes. Turn these influences and strategies into a social media campaign or PSA to share with your peers.

Sexual Feelings and Behavior

Lesson 23.2

Essential Question: What skills can you use to make healthy decisions about your sexuality?

Learning Outcomes

After studying this lesson, you will be able to
- describe early sexual feelings in children and adolescents;
- list the phases of the human sexual response cycle;
- analyze factors that affect a person's sexual behavior;
- explain the physical, emotional, and social impacts of sexual relationships; and
- make responsible decisions about sexual activity.

Key Terms

human sexual response cycle
masturbation
orgasm
sexual history

✓ Warm-Up Activity

You Want to Talk About Sex?

Set Goals Being curious about sex is a normal part of a teen's development. Understanding positive sexual health and practices is important, not only for your adolescent years, but also for your lifetime. Why is it important to talk about this subject? Why do you think some people have a hard time talking about sex? Whom might you need to talk to about sex? If you have a hard time discussing this subject, what might make it easier? Think about answers to these questions and then share your thoughts with a classmate. Then, set three SMART goals for identifying a trusted adult who can answer your questions about sex, developing a healthy relationship, and reaching out when you need to talk.

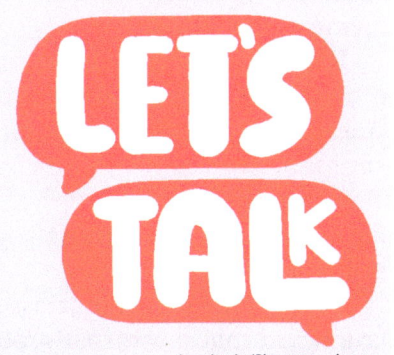
Igor Levin/Shutterstock.com

Sexuality is a natural and important part of human biology and behavior. During puberty, sexual development speeds up. As a result, adolescents experience physical changes and unfamiliar, intense drives and emotions.

It is normal for adolescents to become curious about sex, sexual development, and romantic relationships at this point in their lives. These new thoughts and emotions can be confusing. You probably have questions, which is only natural. Your thoughts, questions, and emotions are the result of human biology unfolding during puberty.

For a happy and healthy transition to adulthood, you need to have reliable information and develop effective skills for dealing with sex, sexuality, and relationships. This lesson should answer some of your questions and help you develop the skills you need to address these important topics.

Early Sexual Feelings

Sexuality is a part of your identity that begins developing long before puberty. In fact, even children experience feelings related to their sexuality and engage in sexual behaviors. From an early age, children are curious about their bodies. Even at a very young age, children may show their genitals to others, touch their genitals for comfort or pleasure, try to look at naked people, or play "doctor" with other children. These actions would be considered inappropriate in older people, but are normal during the development of children.

During the teen years, sexual feelings increase, and people start to become curious about sex. It is normal to feel sexual excitement, or *arousal*, which can be caused by sexual thoughts, daydreams, or images. Teens may find themselves thinking about sex often or having sexual dreams and fantasies about celebrities or people they know. Males may also experience erections and *wet dreams*, or ejaculation that occurs during sleep.

Regardless of biological sex, teens might begin masturbating in response to sexual arousal caused by dreams and fantasies. **Masturbation** is self-stimulation of the reproductive organs and is a common, normal response to sexual excitement. The act of masturbation allows people to safely release sexual tension. During adolescence, masturbation may culminate in orgasm, which you will read about later in this lesson.

Some teens feel embarrassed or guilty about masturbating. They may have heard that masturbation can cause acne, blindness, or other issues. These beliefs are myths. Masturbation does not cause these issues and is a normal, exploratory behavior. Teens who are uncertain about how to respond to sexual excitement can talk about masturbation with a doctor, nurse, parent or guardian, or other trusted adult.

masturbation self-stimulation of the reproductive organs in response to sexual excitement

Human Sexual Response Cycle

During adolescence, many teens experience feelings of sexual attraction. The reproductive organs and brain produce hormones that influence sexual development and these feelings. The combination of romantic and sexual attraction is new, complicated, and intense, but is a normal part of human biology and development.

Sexual attraction often leads to sexual arousal. When a person becomes sexually aroused, physical changes occur in the body. These physical changes progress through four phases: excitement, plateau, orgasm, and resolution. Together, these phases make up the **human sexual response cycle** (**Figure 23.6**).

human sexual response cycle physical changes that occur in the body in response to sexual arousal and activity

Excitement Phase

The excitement phase of sexual response begins with increased blood flow to the sensitive reproductive organs. In females, the clitoris responds by growing longer and swelling. The labia swell, flush with color, and separate. In males, the penis responds by lengthening and hardening.

Sexual stimulation in females causes increased vaginal secretions, which lubricate and prepare the vagina for sexual intercourse. Blood flow increases to the vagina, labia, and clitoris, causing a warm sensation. The breasts swell and become sensitive.

Sexual stimulation in males causes blood to flow into the penis' erectile tissue and results in an erection. The erect penis becomes hard, elongated, and capable of being inserted for sexual intercourse. Heart rate and blood pressure increase in both males and females.

Plateau Phase

During the plateau phase, heart rate and blood pressure continue to rise. In females, blood flow increases to the vaginal wall, the labia continue to swell and flush with color, and the clitoris withdraws under tissue called a *hood*. In males, the penis becomes fully erect, and the testes swell.

Orgasmic Phase

After the plateau phase, sexual excitement may increase and proceed to the orgasmic phase. **Orgasm** is the climax of sexual excitement, characterized by pleasurable sensations in the genital area. This phase is marked by rhythmic muscular contractions in the reproductive organs and throughout the body.

In males, orgasm usually accompanies ejaculation. During ejaculation, muscular contractions forcefully eject semen out of the urethral opening of the penis. Orgasm in females occurs as rhythmic vaginal contractions. Females may also ejaculate fluid from their urethra. During orgasm, males and females experience an intense sense of pleasure and release.

Resolution Phase

During the resolution phase, blood pressure lowers, and heart rate slows down. Less blood flows to the reproductive organs. In females, the labia and clitoris reduce in size and return to their unexcited state. Males lose their erections, and the testes return to their unexcited size and position.

Factors Affecting Sexual Behavior

Many factors influence people's values, views, beliefs, and decisions about sexual behavior. Understanding these factors can help people examine their attitudes about sexual behavior and make healthy decisions.

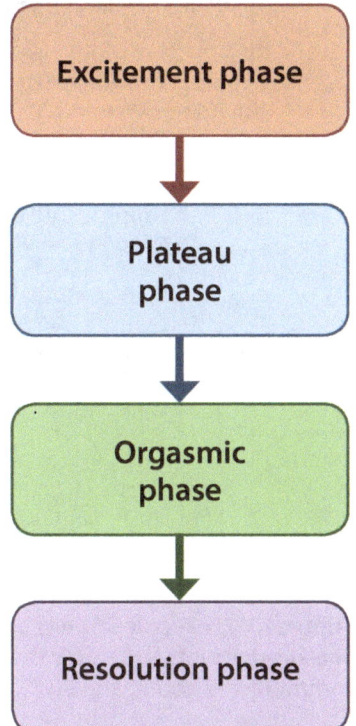

Human Sexual Response Cycle

Figure 23.6 The phases of the human sexual response cycle are accompanied by different physical changes.

orgasm climax of sexual excitement characterized by pleasurable muscular contractions in the reproductive organs and throughout the body

Cultural and Family Background

Different cultures and families have different attitudes regarding sexual behavior and activity (**Figure 23.7**). For example, some cultures see sexual activity as only acceptable in the context of marriage. Other cultures are accepting of sexual activity in committed relationships. Cultures also have varying ideas about what age is appropriate for sexual activity and how openly sexual activity should be discussed. In this way, a person's culture and society shapes opinions and norms regarding sexual activity.

A person's family may also influence attitudes and beliefs. Family members may teach children about the role of sexual activity in a relationship. Through their discussions, they also model for children how sexual activity should be discussed. If sexual activity is treated like a normal part of development, children are more likely to be prepared for handling sexual feelings. If it is not, teens may feel negatively about their sexual feelings and drives.

Many families also have strong beliefs about when sexual activity should begin. These beliefs also influence a person's decisions. For example, teens are more likely to be sexually abstinent if their family members have an unfavorable view of teen sexual activity.

Different cultures and families have differing perspectives on

- the context of appropriate sexual activity (marriage, committed relationship)
- the appropriate age for engaging in sexual activity
- how, when, and with whom sexual activity should be discussed
- the role sexual activity plays in a relationship

Figure 23.7 People's family and cultural backgrounds influence how they value, communicate about, and engage in sexual activity.

Family and Peer Relationships

Teens' relationships have a significant influence on the decisions they make about sexual activity. One important influence is the quality of these relationships. Teens with positive, stable family relationships are less likely to be sexually active. This is also the case for teens with positive, healthy peer relationships. Lower-quality relationships increase the chance a teen will choose to be sexually active.

Relationships also influence what teens perceive as norms surrounding sexual activity. If teens think their peers are sexually active, they are more likely to be sexually active themselves. In reality, however, most teens are not sexually active.

Media

Between social media, music, online videos, and TV, teens use media as many as nine hours per day. This exposure to media can shape a person's values, expectations, attitudes, and behavior. As a result, media with sexual content has an enormous influence on teen sexual activity.

In the US, about 80 percent of TV programs show sexual content, and up to 85 percent of music videos contain sexual or sexually suggestive content. Sexual content in the media often portrays unrealistic and casual attitudes toward sex. Rarely, if ever, do couples in the media discuss their decision to have sex, contraception, or the consequences of sex. These depictions do not reflect the reality of sexual relationships. Sexually explicit media can sometimes show sexual relationships without consent and respect.

Unrealistic or harmful attitudes and expectations can influence people to make unhealthy, uninformed decisions about sexual activity. Fortunately, people can protect themselves from this influence using skills for analyzing and interpreting media messages (**Figure 23.8**). Instead of accepting that media depictions represent reality, teens can question sexual content they see and remember that sexual activity has consequences and many teens are not sexually active.

Goals and Values

Teens who set and work toward clear goals are more likely to avoid risky behaviors, including sexual activity. Clear goals bring into focus the importance of making responsible decisions each day. Each daily, weekly, and monthly decision can impact whether people achieve their goals. For example, having clear goals for the future can make teens less likely to risk the short- and long-term consequences of teen pregnancy or a sexually transmittted infection (STI).

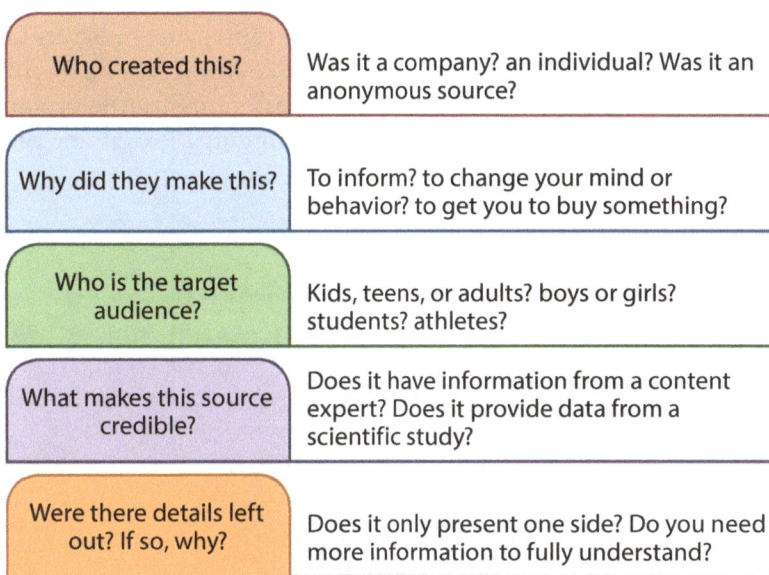

Figure 23.8 Teens can ask specific questions to analyze and interpret media. *What percentage of US TV programs shows sexual content?*

A person's *values*, or what a person considers important, also influence decisions about sexual activity. Values often come from a person's family, culture, society, or education. They guide decisions and behaviors throughout life. Teens who understand their own values are better able to make healthy decisions and are less likely to be pressured into risky behaviors.

Consequences of Sexual Relationships

Sexual activity has many effects on each person in a romantic relationship. The consequences of sexual activity are physical, emotional, and social and can last for a person's lifetime.

Physical Consequences

Sexual activity can have many long-lasting physical consequences. These consequences can alter a person's goals and future decisions and opportunities. Having vaginal sex even once, and even for the first time, can lead to pregnancy and the birth of a baby. As you have learned, becoming a teen parent changes a person's life dramatically and can lead to health conditions for the pregnant person and baby.

Sexual activity of any kind puts people at risk for STIs. Because some STIs are asymptomatic, some people do not know they have an STI. Even so, STIs can lead to infertility and other health conditions. While some are easily treated, others stay for the rest of a person's life.

Emotional Consequences

Just as hormones direct the development of the reproductive system during puberty, they also influence emotions and behavior during and after sexual activity. The hormone *oxytocin* is released by the brain during several different situations, including in-person conversations, holding hands, hugging, sexual activity and orgasm, labor and childbirth, and breastfeeding.

Health in the Media

Portrayal of Sex in the Media

TV shows, movies, music videos, and music use sexual images to get their audience interested and keep them watching. The aim of these images is to entertain, not to educate. As a result, portrayals of sex in the media are often fiction. These portrayals do not show the communication that is part of healthy sexual relationships.

Sometimes, the media can even spread potentially destructive messages about sex. For example, some media portrayals treat people as objects for sexual activity. Others associate sexual activity with aggressive behavior or violence. Media portrayals can also reinforce gender stereotypes and normalize teen sexual activity.

All of these factors can have negative influences on how teens view sexual activity. Media portrayals that normalize unhealthy behaviors can harm health, and teens may develop unrealistic expectations about sexual relationships. Controlling media exposure and analyzing media messages can help teens manage this influence and make healthy decisions.

 Practice Your Skills

Analyze Influences

View a music video or popular TV show that features young adults or teens. Evaluate the video or show according to the following statements. Use a chart like the one shown to decide whether each statement about sexual behavior is *true* of the video or *false* of the video. Then answer the questions that follow.

After evaluating the music video or TV show, create a blog post or video in which you answer the following questions:

- What were the results of your evaluation? Based on these results, does the video or show you chose have a *realistic* or *unrealistic* portrayal of sex? Why?
- Think about the sexual or romantic situations in the music video or TV show. How do these differ from your real-life experiences?
- Is there anything wrong with portraying people as sexual objects? How do these portrayals affect people's behavior? Explain.
- Do you think the images and messages in the video or show you chose influence teens' views about sex? If so, how? Explain your answer.

Statement	True?	False?
People are portrayed as objects for sexual activity.		
People often wear revealing clothes.		
People's physical appearances seem more important than other personal qualities.		
Kissing and sexual activity are important parts of the story or plot.		
Most of the dialogue focuses on discussions about sexual relationships or sexual activity.		
Most scenes that portray romantic relationships show or imply sexual activity.		
People assume (do not actively seek) consent for sexual activity.		
Abstinence or contraceptive use is not shown, implied, or discussed.		

Skills for Health and Wellness

Use the Decision-Making Process: Sexual Activity

Decisions about sexual activity can be difficult to make, especially if you feel pressured or feel like everyone around you is having sex. In hard decisions like this one, it is especially important to use decision-making skills and follow the decision-making process.

You learned about the six steps of the decision-making process in Chapter 2. Following is an example of how you could apply it to a situation where someone is asking you to have sex.

Using the Decision-Making Process: Sexual Activity

Step 1: Define the decision or problem.	You know you do not want to have sex, but your partner keeps asking you. In the past, you have just ignored your partner's question and changed the subject. You need to make a decision about how you will remain abstinent in this situation.
Step 2: Explore alternatives and options.	With a friend, you brainstorm ways of handling the situation. You think of the following alternatives: • Wait until your partner gives up on asking you. • Change your mind about waiting to have sex. • Use your refusal skills the next time your partner asks you. • Start a conversation with your partner about your views on sex. • End the dating relationship.
Step 3: Consider the consequences.	You work on identifying the potential consequences of each alternative. Waiting until your partner stops asking might ruin your relationship, and ending the relationship will mean not dating your partner anymore. Changing your mind will compromise your values. Using refusal skills will work, but it might be easier to start the conversation ahead of time instead of waiting until your partner next wants to have sex.
Step 4: Identify the best alternative.	You choose to start a conversation with your partner. It is time to discuss both of your views about sex.
Step 5: Decide and act.	You put your decision into action by telling your partner you want to meet up and talk about something. You practice what you want to say ahead of time with your friend.
Step 6: Evaluate and revise.	After talking with your partner, your partner seems surprised, but will respect your decision. You decide to use refusal skills if your partner asks again. If your partner tries to pressure you, you will end the dating relationship.

 Practice Your Skills

Make Decisions

What tough decisions do teens in your school have to make about sex? Think about this question and then write a realistic case study about a teen facing a difficult decision related to sex. For example, the teen in your story could be debating whether to be sexually abstinent or trying to get real answers to questions about sex. After writing your case study, place it in a pile with the case studies of your classmates. Choose another classmate's case study at random and read it.

Now, use the decision-making process to help the teen in the case study you chose make the decision or solve the problem. Go through each step of the decision-making process and explain how the teen makes the decision. Complete the case study with the outcome of the decision and then return the case study to the person who wrote it. Assess the decision made in the case study you wrote. Would you have made a different decision? Explain.

Oxytocin, often called the *cuddling hormone*, also affects the brain by causing sensations of bonding, closeness, and nurturing. Sometimes, these sensations can be very intense. Most teens are not ready to handle the intense emotions associated with a sexual relationship like jealousy or vulnerability. Many teens may feel overwhelmed by these new emotions. Teens may also have to cope with the stress of a possible pregnancy or STI. After forming an intimate bond, a couple will have a harder time after a breakup.

Social Consequences

Teens who have a sexual relationship may face unexpected social consequences. Sometimes peers view sexually active teens negatively. Sexual activity can also cause conflict in family relationships if family members disapprove of teens' decisions.

When teen couples become sexually active, they often spend more time together and less time with other friends. This can harm friendships and other relationships. Friends who disapprove of teen sexual relationships may avoid the couple, leaving them isolated.

Making Decisions About Sex

According to experts, the most responsible decision teens can make related to sexual activity is *sexual abstinence*. Sexual abstinence involves refraining from sexual activity. Its benefits, which you learned about in Lesson 14.5, include protection from pregnancy and STIs, emotional maturity, time for personal growth and relationships, and greater enjoyment of nonsexual activities. Abstinence can be hard to practice, but will help you protect your health, relationships, and future dreams and goals.

When making decisions about sex, couples should be able to discuss sex openly (**Figure 23.9**). Both partners should carefully consider their values, their goals for the future, and the risks associated with sex. During this conversation, couples should do the following:

- *Discuss* their views on sex and ways to handle STIs or an unplanned pregnancy. This discussion should occur early in the relationship, before people become sexually involved or aroused. Both partners should be able to give their views openly and honestly, knowing their partner will listen and understand. If a person is undecided about sex, that person should make a decision before beginning a romantic relationship. It takes maturity to share, communicate honestly, and trust.
- *Respect* the other person's decision about sex. Partners must respect each other's commitment to sexual abstinence. Before having sex, each partner must consent to sex. One person cannot make the decision for the other person or assume the other person will go along.
- *Agree* on the methods for carrying out the decision. If the couple decides to be sexually abstinent, they should discuss how they will stick to that decision. Couples who are sexually active should agree on methods for preventing pregnancy and STIs. You will learn more about methods for preventing pregnancy in Chapter 24.
- *Share* information about their **sexual history**, or past sexual activity and partners. If either partner has an STI, the couple must discuss this and take steps to prevent transmission.

sexual history information about a person's past sexual activity and partners

Openly and honestly discuss views on sex

You should know your views on sex before engaging in a sexual relationship.

Respect each other's decisions about sex

Each person should respect their partner's decision to practice sexual abstinence and only engage in sex if both people consent.

Agree on the methods for carrying out the decision

Methods for maintaining abstinence or preventing pregnancies and STIs should be decided together.

Share information about sexual history

Talk to each other about past sexual activity and partners, including any history of STIs.

Figure 23.9 If teens do not know their views on sex and cannot talk openly and honestly with their partner about sex, they are not be ready to have a sexual relationship.

Lesson 23.2 Review

Know and Understand
1. What happens during orgasm in males and females?
2. How does family background influence a teen's decisions about sexual activity?
3. Why are sexual relationships more emotionally intense than relationships without sexual activity?
4. What is the most responsible decision teens can make related to sexual activity?

Think Critically
5. Why is masturbation a safer release of sexual tension than teen sexual activity?
6. Why do you think high-quality relationships make teens less likely to engage in sexual activity?
7. What unrealistic expectations about sexual activity have you seen media depictions set?
8. Why is it important for couples to share their sexual histories before becoming sexually active?

REAL WORLD Health Skills

Access Information When it comes to sex, people sometimes say that "everyone is doing it." The media may support this belief by portraying teens and young adults involved in casual sexual relationships with no responsibilities attached. Using reliable and valid resources, research the latest statistics on teens and sexual activity. How many teens are actually sexually active? Are these sexual relationships truly casual, with no responsibilities attached? Record a short video, podcast episode, or PSA discussing the phrase "everyone is doing it."

Chapter 23 Review and Assessment

Chapter Summary

Sexuality is a part of identity that includes your biological sex, gender identity and expression, sexual orientation, and sexual experiences and thoughts. Biological sex describes whether you are genetically and physically male or female. Biological sex is often assigned at birth, but can be ambiguous. In contrast, gender describes the characteristics society associates with a biological sex.

Society often assumes particular gender roles and stereotypes. Gender stereotypes can harm self-esteem and a person's relationships, especially since people do not exhibit only masculine or feminine traits. Gender identity refers to a person's deeply held, internal thoughts and feelings about gender. People who are gender nonconforming have a gender identity that does not match their biological sex. People who are nonbinary have a gender that falls outside the categories of man or woman.

Sexual orientation is a person's enduring pattern of romantic and/or sexual attraction to others. People use many different words to describe sexual and romantic orientation. Often, people who are gender nonconforming or have a nonheterosexual orientation identify as LGBT+. People who are LGBT+ may face discrimination. Being an upstander and advocating for safe zones can help these people feel accepted.

Sexual feelings increase during the teen years, and people start to become curious about sex. Some teens may feel sexual excitement, or arousal. Some may have sexual fantasies or wet dreams. Teens might masturbate in response to this arousal. Physical changes in the body during sexual arousal are called the human sexual response cycle and include the following phases: excitement, plateau, orgasm, and resolution.

Sexuality develops over a person's lifetime, starting in childhood. Many factors affect sexual behavior, including cultural and family background, relationships, media, and goals and values. Sexual relationships have lasting physical, emotional, and social consequences. Therefore, it is important to make responsible decisions about sex and discuss this decision with a partner. Making wise decisions about sex is part of promoting personal health.

Vocabulary Activity

Imagine you want to have a conversation with a trusted adult about one of the topics in this chapter. Write a script in which you have this conversation, using the key terms shown appropriately. Express your thoughts and feelings, as well as what you believe the trusted adult's thoughts and feelings would be. After writing the script, reflect on what you have written. Why is it important to use these key terms accurately? How could you educate people who do not know them about their meanings?

cisgender	*homophobia*	*orgasm*
disorder of sex development (DSD)	*human sexual response cycle*	*same-sex marriage*
		sexual history
gender binary	*LGBT+*	*sexuality*
gender identity	*masturbation*	*sexual orientation*
gender nonconforming	*nonbinary*	*transgender*

Review and Recall

Review the information in this chapter by answering the following questions.

1. What is the difference between gender identity and sexual orientation?
2. Which chromosome combination results in a biological male? biological female?

3. What does it mean to be born with a disorder of sex development (DSD)?
4. Which of the following is *not* an aspect of sexuality?
   A. sexual orientation
   B. hormonal balance
   C. biological sex
   D. sexual experiences
5. When do sexually ambiguous traits begin to appear in children with Turner Syndrome or Klinefelter Syndrome?
6. Which term describes people who identify with the gender opposite their biological, anatomical sex?
   A. bisexual
   B. heterosexual
   C. homosexual
   D. transgender
7. What defines expectations for masculinity and femininity?
   A. society
   B. nature
   C. birth
   D. biological sex
8. Which hormone is often called the *cuddling hormone* and affects the brain by causing sensations of bonding, closeness, and nurturing?
9. What are the four phases in the human sexual response cycle?
10. During which phase of the human sexual response cycle do heart rate and blood pressure continue to rise?
    A. excitement
    B. plateau
    C. orgasm
    D. resolution
11. What is the climax of sexual excitement?
    A. orgasm
    B. masturbation
    C. arousal
    D. plateau
12. What is one thing couples should discuss when making decisions about sex?
13. What is another term for sexual excitement?
    A. wet dream
    B. masturbation
    C. arousal
    D. orgasm

Standardized Test Prep

Reading and Writing Practice

Read the passage below and then answer the following questions.

> The phrase "coming out" is short for "coming out of the closet." When people who are LGBT+ come out, they are telling their family members, friends, and others about this part of their identity.
>
> Coming out can be scary, especially if family members or friends do not seem accepting. Coming out, however, can be empowering and help people embrace their identities and develop closer, more honest relationships. It can also help a person connect with the larger LGBT+ community and be a role model for others. This can help debunk stereotypes and myths and educate others.
>
> Generally, the process of coming out begins with coming out to one's self. Then it involves coming out to others.

14. Which statement best describes the main point of this passage?
    A. People who are LGBT+ should always come out.
    B. Coming out is scary for many people.
    C. People need to be educated about LGBT+ issues.
    D. Coming out has many benefits for people who are LGBT+ and others.
15. What is the first stage in coming out?
16. The phrase "coming out" is short for what other phrase?

Chapter 23 Skills Assessment

Critical Thinking Skills

Answer the following questions to assess your knowledge of what you learned in this chapter.

1. What is the advantage of allowing individuals with DSDs to select their gender when they grow up? Do you think a person should be required to select a gender?
2. Is developing a "crush" on a member of the same sex always an expression of homosexuality in an adolescent? Why or why not?
3. Does your school have an LGBT+ support group? If not, do you think one is needed? With a partner, brainstorm some steps you could take to start one.
4. What can be done to help teens who are unsure about their gender identities or sexual orientations?
5. Do you think the term LGBT+ is an adequate and accurate term? Why or why not? Can you think of a better term? Explain your answer.
6. What does the term homophobia mean to you? In what ways have you seen it displayed?
7. How can you respect other people's views on sexuality, even if they differ from your own?
8. Is gender identity chosen or assigned? Explain your answer.
9. With a partner, discuss several examples of inaccurate depictions of sex in the media. What are some ways you can protect yourself from unrealistic views of sexual activity presented in the media?
10. How might a sexually active relationship affect other relationships?
11. What might prevent romantic partners from discussing their views on sex?
12. What are some examples of situations that might make sexual abstinence difficult?
13. Make a list of questions you have about sex. Then, create an action plan to help you consult reliable sources and trusted adults for the answers to your questions.

Health and Wellness Skills

Complete the following activities to assess your skills related to health and wellness.

14. **Analyze Influences.** Think about all of the factors that influence your sexual behaviors and decisions. What factors do you think have had a positive influence on your sexual behaviors and decisions? Describe examples. What factors have had a negative influence? Describe these as well. What strategies could you use to avoid the negative factors and increase the positive?
15. **Access Information.** Learning about sex from unreliable sources can lead teens to believe myths and misconceptions about sex. Research places you could go to get credible, reliable, and valid information about topics related to sex. These places may be online or in your community. Create an infographic or one-page handout listing the resources you found and describing what makes them credible, reliable, and valid.
16. **Make Decisions.** Making the decision to remain sexually abstinent can be difficult, but can prevent many health risks. Write down five factors you should consider before making this decision. Are these factors strong enough for you to stick with your decision to remain sexually abstinent? Are there some considerations you could focus on that would help you remain abstinent? Underline the strong considerations and cross out the weak ones. Add any additional considerations that are strong considerations.
17. **Set Goals.** Gender roles and stereotypes can cause confusion and strain for people and their relationships. With a partner, discuss how gender roles and stereotypes influence you. Then, create three SMART goals to help you navigate gender roles and stereotypes and promote an environment that is respectful of gender diversity. Act on one of these goals and evaluate how it influences you personally and those around you.

18. **Communicate with Others.** Imagine your school has an anonymous hotline where students can call in for advice about different situations. You are a member of the student group trained to answer these calls and provide advice. You answer a call from a student who is questioning personal gender identity and sexual orientation. What would you say to this student to encourage healthy thoughts and help the person open a line of communication with a trusted adult?

19. **Practice Health-Enhancing Behaviors.** Although sexual abstinence is the most responsible decision for teens, some teens make the decision to become sexually active. If teens decide to be sexually active, what are some factors these teens should talk about with each other to try and reduce the associated risks? Create a journal entry that discusses these factors. Consider how these factors could also affect a future sexual relationship during adulthood.

20. **Advocate for Health.** Research and define the term *homophobia*. What views does homophobia include? Do these views exist in your community? in your school? In small groups, list some examples of homophobia, including physical, mental, emotional, sexual, and verbal abuse or bullying and cyberbullying. Next, discuss actions you could take to help someone experiencing these types of bullying. As a group, come up with a positive message that could take the place of the homophobic message. Share your work with the class.

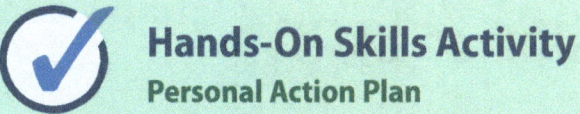

Hands-On Skills Activity
Personal Action Plan

In this chapter, and in other chapters, you have learned about healthy teen relationships, the risks of being sexually active as a teen, and the benefits of remaining sexually abstinent. In this activity, you will formulate a *Personal Action Plan* you can use when faced with challenges to your own sexual values and decisions.

Steps for This Activity

1. On a separate sheet of paper or electronically, create a chart as described in the following steps.
2. **Set Goals.** Consider your current goals and dreams. In a box labeled *Now*, list your short-term goals. Where do you hope to be in one year? What are your current dreams and hobbies? What do you enjoy about your life? In a box labeled *Later*, list your long-term goals and dreams. Where do you hope to be in 10 years? What do you want your life to look like? What do you want to achieve?
3. Explore your own personal values. What beliefs are important to you and why? Could you defend these values and beliefs, if challenged? How do these values and beliefs fit into your present and future goals and dreams? How do your values and beliefs affect your sexual behavior and your reaction to challenges of a sexual nature? At the bottom of your chart, list your most important values and beliefs and how they relate to challenges of a sexual nature.
4. **Practice Health-Enhancing Behaviors.** In boxes between *Now* and *Later*, formulate pledges or promises to yourself that will help you reach your *Later* goals. These pledges are personal oaths or statements you can use when faced with sexual challenges. The pledges could range from not drinking alcohol or using drugs, to only kissing, to communicating your consent, boundaries, and wishes to your partner. As you formulate these pledges, think about the different challenging situations you might face. How far would you be willing to go sexually if someone asked you? How might alcohol, drugs, or being in a bedroom affect your decisions?
5. When complete, keep your *Personal Action Plan* in a place where you can reference it or change it, if needed.

Chapter 24: Pregnancy Prevention

Lesson 24.1   What Is Contraception?
Lesson 24.2   Barrier Methods
Lesson 24.3   Hormonal Methods
Lesson 24.4   Natural Methods and Sterilization

Look for the skills icon throughout this chapter for opportunities to practice your health skills.

Check Your Health and Wellness Skills

In this chapter, you will learn skills for preventing pregnancy. To understand the skills you currently use, take the following inventory of your behaviors. Indicate how well you think you use each skill. Use a scale of 1–5, *1* meaning you do not use the skill and *5* meaning you feel completely comfortable using it.

Skill	How Well Do You Use Each Skill?
I know where to get reliable information about contraception.	
I verify the things I hear people saying about contraception before I believe them.	
I feel comfortable discussing my boundaries and consent about contraception with a dating partner.	
I enforce my boundaries and know how to say *no* if someone asks me to cross them.	
I follow the directions on devices and medications exactly.	
I think of and ask questions if I don't understand how to use a device or medication.	
I compare the effectiveness, pros, and cons of devices and medications before purchasing them.	
I have people to go to for advice if I decide to use contraception.	
I understand the importance of using contraception correctly every time.	
I can differentiate between contraceptive methods that are effective or ineffective.	
	Total:

Add up your responses to each statement. The higher your score, the more comfortable you feel preventing pregnancy. Which skill do you think is most important for you? Which skill is the most challenging for you? Which skill would you most like to improve? In this chapter, you will learn how to perform these skills better and more often.

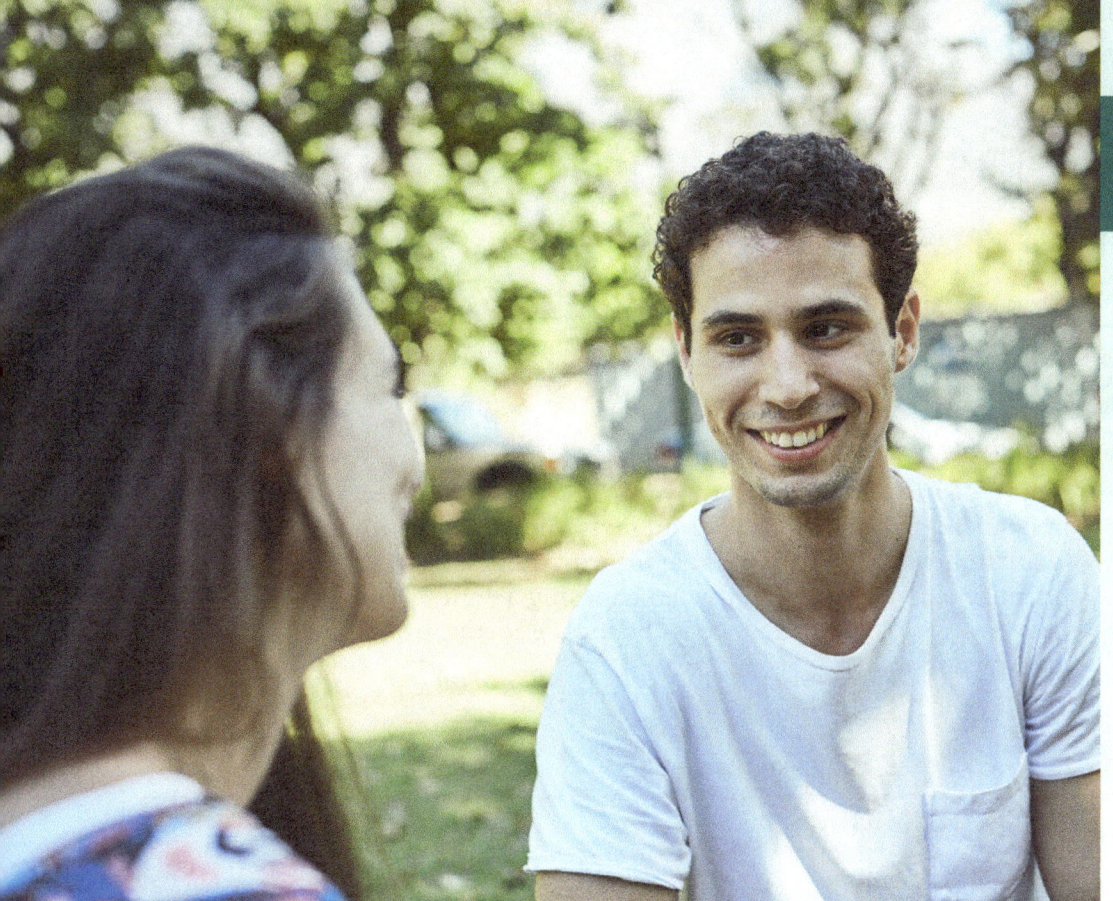
RapidEye/E+/Getty Images

Reading and Notetaking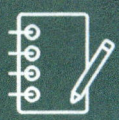

Before reading this chapter, write 12 statements describing what you already know about pregnancy prevention and contraceptive methods. List these statements in a graphic organizer like the one shown. As you read this chapter, decide whether each statement is accurate or not. Add key information from the chapter to your organizer, writing notes as statements. After reading, read your statements aloud with a partner. Check each other's statements for correct spelling, grammar, and pronunciation and revise as needed.

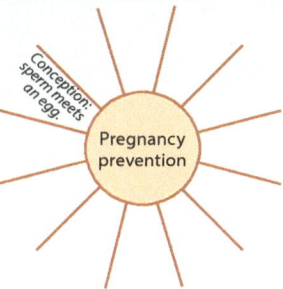

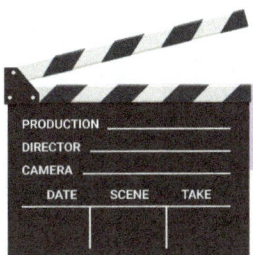

Setting the Scene

Any Risk Is Too Big

You have been dating your partner for nine months. You love your partner and hope you will stay together after high school. Sometimes, you dream about marrying your partner. You often think you have found "the one."

So far in your relationship, you and your partner have decided to be sexually abstinent. Sticking to this decision has been getting harder recently. The other day, your partner said maybe it was time to reconsider the decision. "Contraceptives prevent pregnancy, and some even prevent STIs," your partner said. You love and want to feel close to your partner, but are also nervous. You have a lot of big, long-term goals for your life. You want absolutely no risk for pregnancy.

Thinking Critically

1. Should teens worry about pregnancy, even if they are using contraceptives? Why or why not?
2. What do you think is the most effective way for teens to prevent pregnancy?
3. In this scenario, how could you explain your feelings to your partner clearly and respectfully? What reliable resources could you use to get facts about the effectiveness of contraception?

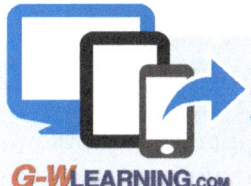

Click on the activity icon or visit www.g-wlearning.com/health/4330 to access online vocabulary activities using key terms from the chapter.

Lesson 24.1 What Is Contraception?

Essential Question?
What is the purpose of contraception, and what is the most effective method?

Key Terms
- barrier methods
- contraception
- hormonal methods
- natural methods
- sterilization

Learning Outcomes

After studying this lesson, you will be able to
- define *contraception*;
- recognize pregnancy prevention facts and myths;
- explain how to identify reliable information about sexual health;
- identify factors to consider when choosing a contraceptive method; and
- assess why sexual abstinence is the most effective method of contraception.

✓ Warm-Up Activity

What Do You Know?

Comprehend Concepts You may have heard the term *contraception* in the media or in your own family. What does the term mean to you? What specifically comes to mind when you hear the term *contraception*? What does *sexual abstinence* mean to you? What do you think are some possible benefits of remaining sexually abstinent? Write a paragraph containing your answers to these questions.

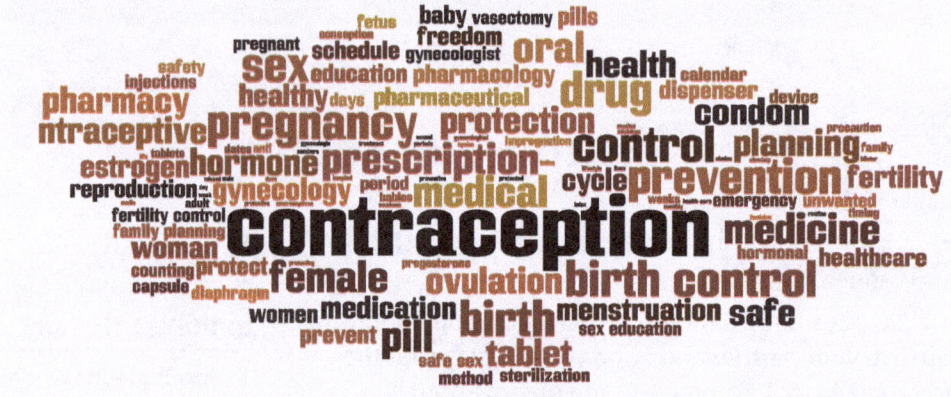

Boris15/Shutterstock.com

Many young people dream of someday having their own families. Parents know, however, that pregnancy and family life demand attention, money, time, and emotional maturity. For people who want to delay having children or do not want children, **contraception** helps prevent pregnancy. It also allows people to remain childless if they choose.

What would you say if a friend asked you how to prevent pregnancy? if you heard someone say pregnancy could be prevented by urinating or douching after sex? How would you react if your dating partner told you pregnancy was not possible the first time you had sex?

contraception any method that reduces the risk of pregnancy resulting from sexual activity

As your peers talk about sexuality and sex, you have probably heard many misconceptions or myths. Unfortunately, false information about pregnancy prevention can have serious consequences. Not knowing the facts about contraception can lead to an unplanned pregnancy, now during adolescence or in your adult future. In this chapter, you will learn the facts about contraception, including common types and how to use them.

Health in the Media

Media Messages About Contraception

Some teens spend fewer hours in school than they do using some form of media, including TV shows, online videos, music, and social media. Most media content is entertainment and is not trying to share reliable information. As a result, teens consume a lot of media containing mixed messages, unrealistic situations, and untrue information.

Because sexual activity is common in media portrayals, teens are exposed to a lot of unrealistic information about sex and contraception. For example, most movies with sexual content do not show or discuss the consequences of sexual activity, such as pregnancy and STIs. Most movies also have no information about contraception and show people engaging in sexual activity without even discussing pregnancy prevention.

Movies also commonly depict sexual activity involving people who do not discuss the decision to have sex, consent, contraception, or the potential consequences of sex. In fact, it is unusual for movies to show *any* serious consequences of sex.

As a result of these representations, teens may not realize discussing contraception and STI prevention is an essential part of having a healthy sexual relationship. Teens may think talking about contraception is unromantic or interrupts the mood. In reality, discussing contraception is a way of showing care and respect and protecting both partners from the potentially negative consequences of sex.

 Practice Your Skills

Advocate for Health

Think about the movies, books, TV shows, online videos, and music you have seen, read, or listened to in the past six months. Which of these forms of media contained sexual content? List all the media that contained sexual content and then assess each one using the following criteria. Tally how often the statements were true or false of the media you consumed. Then, in a group, discuss how often the statements were true or false. How do you think these messages affect teens? Create an alternative, realistic, health-enhancing message for each statement. Make sure your statements appeal to your target audience: teens. Share these messages with your peers.

Media Message	True	False	Alternative Realistic Message
Having sex once can't cause pregnancy.			
Adults are not worried about becoming pregnant.			
Having sex has no negative consequences.			
People don't talk about using contraception before having sex.			
Having casual sex has no negative consequences.			
You don't have to worry about STIs when you have sex.			

Myths and Facts About Pregnancy Prevention

Many myths exist about how pregnancy occurs and can be prevented. Believing these myths can have life-changing consequences. The best way to guard against myths is to learn the facts about contraception and pregnancy and evaluate sources carefully (**Figure 24.1**). Following are some common myths and facts about pregnancy prevention:

Myth #1: A female who urinates after sex will not get pregnant.
Fact: Urinating after sex does *not* prevent pregnancy.

Myth #2: Douching, or cleaning the inside of the vagina, after sex prevents pregnancy.
Fact: Douching after sex does *not* prevent pregnancy. In fact, douching can increase the likelihood of pregnancy by pushing semen deeper into the vagina. Douching also does not prevent the transmission of STIs and HIV.

Myth #3: Pregnancy cannot occur the first time people have sex.
Fact: Someone *can* become pregnant the first time people have sex. Having sex or using contraception that is not 100 percent effective can lead to pregnancy and STI transmission any time people have sex, including the first time.

Myth #4: A female cannot become pregnant while menstruating.
Fact: Females *can* become pregnant during menstruation. It is unlikely, but possible. Females with regular menstrual cycles of 28–32 days will typically not become pregnant during menstruation. Many females, however, have irregular periods. Some have shorter cycles (24 days, for example), and some ovulate earlier than the 14th day. These people can become pregnant during menstruation.

Myth #5: Pregnancy cannot occur if the male withdraws, or "pulls out," before ejaculating.
Fact: Someone *can* become pregnant even if a male withdraws before ejaculation. Often, the penis releases some fluid containing sperm before ejaculation. *Withdrawal*, covered later in this chapter, is the least effective method of contraception.

Myth #6: Pregnancy will not occur if someone stands up during or after sex.
Fact: People *can* become pregnant no matter the position during and after sex. Standing up during or after sex will not prevent pregnancy.

Myth #7: A female younger than 18 years of age cannot become pregnant.
Fact: Females younger than 18 years of age can and do become pregnant. Someone who has begun menstruating can become pregnant regardless of age.

Evaluating Information About Sexual Health	
Ask Yourself	**Why?**
Does the source have medical expertise?	Because contraception is based on anatomy and physiology, sources should have medical and scientific expertise. For example, a reliable source might be a medical organization, such as the Mayo Clinic, a hospital and research facility. The Mayo Clinic employs doctors with MD degrees and expert researchers with PhD or MS degrees.
What is the mission or objective of the source?	An organization's website should list its mission, or purpose and goals. A reliable source is dedicated to promoting physical and mental health. Employees should have medical and scientific expertise.
Does the source describe alternatives?	Contraception is complicated. Some methods may not be right for certain people. Therefore, a source should offer several options, and their advantages and disadvantages. This allows people to make a responsible decision.
Is the source a profit-making organization?	Some organizations are businesses with the goal of making money. The information these organizations present may be biased. For example, a company that makes a certain type of contraception may present incomplete or misleading information about abstinence or other contraceptive methods.

Figure 24.1 Asking yourself specific questions can help you verify sources will contain accurate and relevant information for your health.

Myth #8: People will not contract an STI or HIV as long as they use a condom during sexual activity.
Fact: If used properly and consistently, latex, polyurethane, and polyisoprene condoms can reduce—but not eliminate—the risk of contracting an STI or HIV.

Myth #9: Pregnancy is not that common after sex.
Fact: In a given year, 85 out of 100 females who have sex without contraception will become pregnant. If you have sex without contraception, you only have a 15 percent chance of *not* getting pregnant.

Myth #10: Pregnancy will not occur if people use contraception during sex.
Fact: Using contraception reduces, but does not eliminate, the risk of pregnancy. The chance of becoming pregnant depends on the contraceptive method used. Some methods are more effective than others. The risk of pregnancy also depends on whether people use contraception consistently and correctly. Abstinence is the *only* way to avoid pregnancy completely.

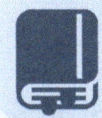

Case Study

Is That Really True?

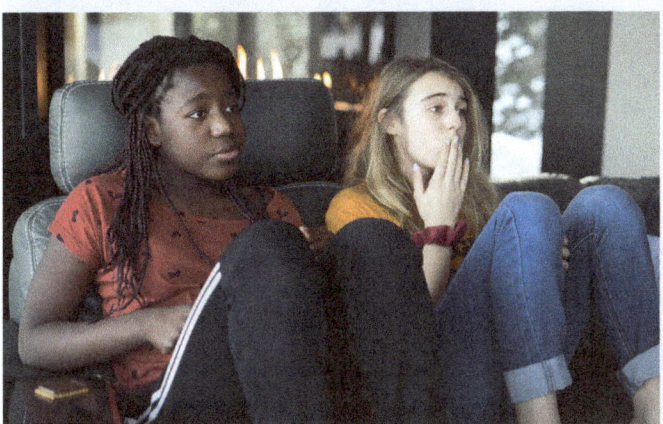

marieclaudelemay/iStock / Getty Images Plus/Getty Images

Raegan was scrolling through social media when she came across an article claiming she cannot become pregnant while on her period. Raegan knows you cannot believe everything you see online and she does not think this sounds right. Raegan also recognizes this article is not a credible source of health information. She is not completely sure, however. Raegan wants to find reliable information about this claim, but does not know where to look.

Sitting at home, Jayden overhears his older brother's conversation on the phone. His older brother says, "Condoms and birth control are such a hassle. Why doesn't he just pull out? Problem solved." Jayden knows his brother is wrong. Pulling out is not that effective and does not protect against STIs. He does not know if it is his place to correct his brother. At the same time, he worries his brother will spread this misinformation if he says nothing.

One night, Sonja was watching her favorite show with her best friend. During the show, two characters had sex, and the female character was worried about becoming pregnant since they did not use a condom. The male character told her, "Don't worry. It was only one time. You won't get pregnant." Sonja's friend scoffed at this, and Sonja was confused. Was the male character wrong?

Practice Your Skills

Make Decisions

In these scenarios, each teen has a decision to make about how to get reliable information or share that information with others. Using the decision-making process, complete one scenario to show how the teen gets factual information or corrects a myth. Explain how the teen completes each step of the decision-making process. Have the teen go back and revise the decision if it does not work. Then, share the factual information the teen found with the class and cite your sources.

barrier methods
contraceptive methods that prevent sperm from traveling through the female reproductive system and fertilizing an egg

hormonal methods
contraceptive methods that alter a person's hormone levels to thicken cervical mucus and inhibit ovulation (the release of an egg)

natural methods
contraceptive methods that time sexual activity with a female's menstrual cycle and the sexual response cycle to prevent the sperm and egg from meeting

sterilization contraceptive method that permanently prevents pregnancy by altering the reproductive system, often through surgery

Types of Contraception

There are many contraceptive methods, and people must choose the method that works best for them. People can consult a healthcare professional if they have questions about selecting a method. A healthcare professional and the manufacturer's instructions for the product or device provide information about how to use contraceptives. The main categories of contraceptive methods are

- *sexual abstinence*—is the only 100-percent effective method of preventing pregnancy;
- **barrier methods**—prevent sperm from traveling through the female reproductive system and fertilizing an egg;
- **hormonal methods**—alter a person's hormone levels to thicken cervical mucus and inhibit ovulation;
- **natural methods**—time sexual activity with a female's menstrual cycle and the sexual response cycle; and
- **sterilization**—permanently prevents pregnancy by altering the reproductive system, often through surgery.

You will learn more about each of these methods later in this chapter.

Contraceptive methods are only effective if they are used correctly every single a time a person has sexual intercourse. Not using contraception correctly just one time can lead to pregnancy. If a person forgets to use contraception during sexual intercourse or notices a contraceptive method fails (for example, if a condom breaks), *emergency contraception* can help prevent pregnancy. Emergency contraception does *not* end a pregnancy that has already begun. Instead, it uses hormones to prevent pregnancy from occurring.

Even with contraception, sexual activity is risky, especially during adolescence. Though condoms help protect people against STIs and HIV, other contraceptive methods do not. Only sexual abstinence is 100 percent effective in preventing pregnancy and STIs.

Questions to Consider When Selecting Contraception

- How effective is it in preventing pregnancies?
- Does it also protect against STIs and HIV?
- How easy is it to use? Can you forget to use it or use it incorrectly? Can it break?
- How much does this method cost? What are the up-front costs, and how much will it cost over time?
- Do I need a doctor's prescription for this method?
- Is this method reversible?

Figure 24.2 Different methods of contraception vary in effectiveness, cost, ease of use, and availability. To determine the right method for you, reflect on these questions. *Which category of contraception permanently prevents pregnancy?*

Factors to Consider When Selecting Contraception

Each contraceptive method has advantages and disadvantages (**Figure 24.2**). People should consider their goals, sexual history, and any STIs when selecting a method. Is the goal to prevent pregnancy and have protection from STIs and HIV? Certain methods, such as condoms, can reduce the risk of pregnancy, STIs, and HIV. Other methods, such as hormonal contraception, reduce the risk of pregnancy, but do not protect from STIs and HIV.

People should also consider the cost and availability of contraception. Some methods, such as a condom or spermicide, are inexpensive and can be obtained without a doctor's prescription. Other methods, such as the intrauterine device (IUD), require a doctor's visit. A person using the birth control shot must visit the doctor regularly.

Some people want to use a *reversible* method of contraception so they can choose to have children in the future. Others would prefer a method that is permanent. Sterilization is permanent and practically irreversible. You will learn about sterilization in Lesson 24.4.

Ease of use is another important factor. Each method of contraception is effective only when used correctly every time, which may not always be convenient or possible. Some people cannot use certain types of contraception, such as hormonal methods, because of health conditions or activities like smoking.

Skills for Health and Wellness

Answering Questions About Your Sexual Health

Many teens have questions about their sexual health and contraception. Turning to unreliable sources for answers or believing myths can have negative consequences and lead to pregnancy. It is best to get answers using reliable resources, such as credible websites, books, or magazines; healthcare professionals; or other trusted adults. Different people prefer to use different resources, depending on their level of comfort and relationships. Learning how to answer these important questions will help you protect your health now and into adulthood.

 Practice Your Skills

Access Information

What is one question you have related to sexual health or contraception? Be specific about what you want to know. Then get a factual answer by accessing reliable information. For this activity, try to find your answer online. Use the following steps:

1. Start by searching for online resources that answer your question. Use search terms that clearly relate to your question.
2. Visit websites with reliable information. If possible, navigate directly to a website you know is reliable. For example, you could visit the website of a professional health organization like the ones that follow and search for an answer there.

Sources for Information About Adolescent Sexual Health	
American Academy of Pediatrics	www.aap.org
American Sexual Health Association	www.ashasexualhealth.org
Center for Young Women's Health	www.youngwomenshealth.org
Centers for Disease Control and Prevention	www.cdc.gov
Mayo Clinic	www.mayoclinic.org
US Department of Health and Human Services	www.healthfinder.gov
Young Men's Health	www.youngmenshealthsite.org

3. To evaluate whether a website is reliable, ask the following questions:
   - What is the URL stem? Websites ending with .org, .gov, or .edu are most reliable. Websites ending with .com are usually business or commercial and may be making money related to the information they provide.
   - Does the website advertise products or belong to a business that sells products? You cannot trust websites that are trying to sell products or services.
   - Who is the author or sponsor of the website? Do not rely on opinion articles, editorials, or blogs. Use websites and articles authored by someone with medical expertise from the professional healthcare or health science field.
   - Does the website cite specific scientific studies to support its information?
   - Is the source current? Progress in science and technology can make information out of date.
4. Check the information you find against other sources. You should be able to find the same facts from other reliable sources, such as professional health organization or hospital websites. You could also check your information with a doctor or other healthcare professional.

After getting an answer to your question, create a social media post, blog post, or journal entry explaining the answer. Be sure to cite your sources.

Sometimes, people have strong preferences and views about contraception. Fortunately, the least expensive method of preventing pregnancy is also the most effective: sexual abstinence.

Abstinence: The Most Effective Method of Contraception

There is only one 100 percent effective method of preventing pregnancy, and that is sexual abstinence. Abstinence is also 100 percent effective at protecting against STIs. In addition, abstinence has other social and emotional benefits, which you learned about previously. These benefits include emotional maturity, time for personal growth and relationships, enjoyment of nonsexual activities, and the freedom to pursue one's goals without worrying about pregnancy or STIs.

Abstinence does not involve purchasing devices such as condoms, visiting the doctor for a shot, or taking a pill at the same time every day. Because of this, abstinence costs nothing. It is not expensive like some methods of contraception.

For some people, practicing abstinence can be difficult. People may feel pressured to have sex or get caught up in sexual attraction. By remembering their goals, avoiding risky situations, and using refusal skills, people can face these challenges and stay committed to abstinence. This commitment will help them pursue their goals, build healthy relationships, and prepare for a healthy adulthood.

Lesson 24.1 Review

Know and Understand
1. What is the purpose of contraception?
2. Why is it important to get reliable, factual information about contraception?
3. How are barrier methods different from hormonal methods of contraception?
4. Why is ease of use an important factor when choosing contraception?
5. What advantages does sexual abstinence have over other methods of contraception?

Think Critically
6. List one myth you have heard about contraception. What is the fact that debunks the myth?
7. Why are contraceptive methods only effective if they are used correctly every single time a person has sexual intercourse?

✓ REAL WORLD Health Skills

Set Goals Create a dream board of you and your ideal life in 10 years. Note whether you have a romantic partner or are single. Draw or find pictures of the kind of home, belongings and experiences, and job you want. Where would you like to live? Do you have kids at this point in your life? Now, imagine you are in your senior year and contract an incurable STI or are due to have a child the month you graduate. How would this picture change? Would accomplishing this picture be possible? Would it be harder? Would it take longer? How would being sexually active affect your goals? What short-term goals could you set to make sure you reach your long-term goals?

Barrier Methods

Lesson 24.2

Essential Question: How do barrier methods help prevent pregnancy?

Learning Outcomes

After studying this lesson, you will be able to
- explain how barrier methods reduce the risk of pregnancy;
- list the steps in applying and removing an external condom;
- describe how to apply and remove an internal condom;
- discuss how the contraceptive sponge helps prevent pregnancy;
- understand how to use a diaphragm for contraception; and
- analyze how people use the cervical cap to avoid pregnancy.

Key Terms

cervical cap
contraceptive sponge
diaphragm
spermicide

Warm-Up Activity

Talk About Condoms

Analyze Influences Barrier methods are some of the most common methods of contraception used. As a class, discuss the following question: *What have you heard about condoms?* Share what you have heard about condoms from advertisements, conversations, and media portrayals. List these messages in a chart like the one that follows. Then assess whether you think each message is accurate or not. How do these messages influence teens?

Message	Is It Accurate?	Influence on Teens

Barrier methods are a common type of contraception. These methods physically reduce the risk of fertilization and pregnancy by preventing sperm from reaching the egg inside the female reproductive system. Each barrier method has advantages and disadvantages. For example, condoms protect against STIs and HIV, while other methods do not.

No barrier method is 100 percent effective in preventing pregnancy or STI transmission. For example, even if a person with genital herpes or human papillomavirus (HPV) does not have visible sores, the virus may be present on skin not covered by a condom. The virus can then spread to the person's partner during sexual activity.

Some barrier methods are easier to use than others. Barrier methods of contraception include external condoms, internal condoms, the diaphragm, the cervical cap, and the contraceptive sponge (**Figure 24.3**).

Figure 24.3 To be effective, each method must be used correctly every time a person has sexual intercourse.

Barrier Methods

Method	Use	Requires a Doctor's Visit	Estimated Cost	Number of Pregnancies Expected (per 100 Females)
Diaphragm	A flexible cup inserted into the vagina; blocks sperm from entering the uterus	Yes	$0–$250 (including doctor's visit) depending on insurance	12
Contraceptive sponge	A sponge inserted into the vagina; contains *spermicide* (a chemical that kills sperm) and prevents sperm from entering the uterus	No	$15 for three	12–24
Cervical cap	A silicone cup inserted into the vagina; prevents sperm from entering the uterus	Yes	$0–$275 (including doctor's visit) depending on insurance	14–29
External condom	Fits over an erect penis to block sperm from entering the vagina	No	$2–$6	15
Internal condom	Fits inside the vagina to prevent sperm from entering the uterus	No	$2–$3 each	21
Spermicide	A substance inserted into the vagina that inactivates sperm	No	$8–$15 per kit	28

External Condoms

The *external condom*, sometimes called the *male condom*, is designed to fit over the erect penis during sexual activity. There are several types of external condoms:

- *latex condoms*—made from a form of natural rubber derived from the sap of rubber trees
- *polyurethane condoms*—made from various forms of plastic
- *polyisoprene condoms*—made from synthetic, latex-free rubber
- *natural condoms*—made from the walls of animal intestines; these condoms contain small pores through which pathogens can pass, so they do *not* prevent STIs and HIV

External condoms help prevent pregnancy by catching the semen released during ejaculation and preventing sperm from reaching the egg. In addition, external condoms can be coated with **spermicide**, a substance that inactivates sperm (**Figure 24.4**). An external condom must be applied after an erection and before the penis touches a partner's genitals. This is important because the penis can release fluids containing sperm and possibly pathogens that cause STIs prior to ejaculation. External condoms cannot be reused; a new condom must be used each time intercourse occurs.

Using external condoms has no health-related side effects unless one partner has a latex allergy, which can trigger an allergic reaction if latex condoms are used. People who have a latex allergy should use a different type of condom or a different method of contraception.

External condoms become dry, brittle, and ineffective over time. It is important to check the expiration date and discard expired condoms. People should not store condoms in hot or cold places (like cars) or in wallets, where they can be damaged or punctured. Petroleum-based lotions or lubricants such as Vaseline should not be used with a latex condom. These substances will break down the latex barrier.

Using an external condom is easy, but people should take care to prevent spilling semen. It is a good idea to practice applying and removing a condom before engaging in sexual activity. People can practice by applying an external condom over an object shaped like a penis (**Figure 24.5**).

spermicide substance that inactivates sperm

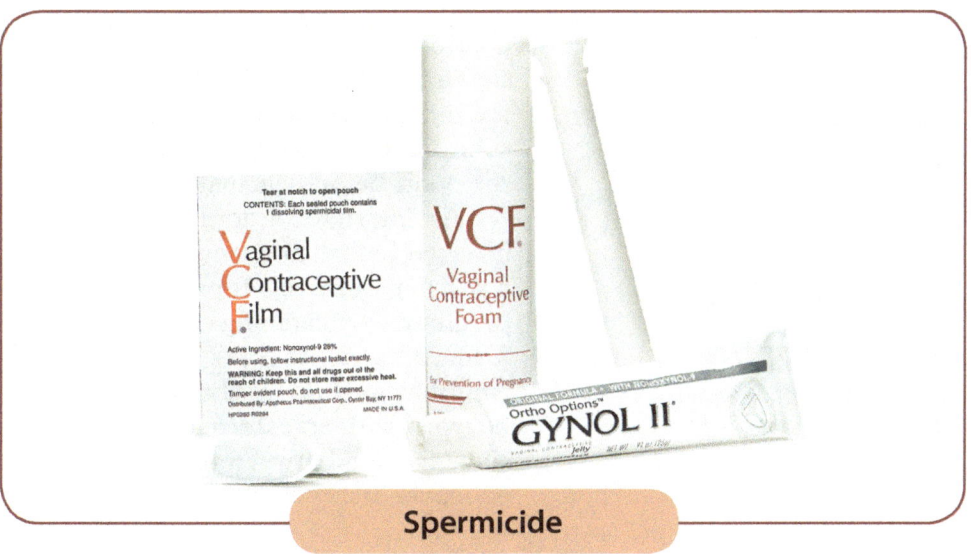

Figure 24.4 Spermicide can also be inserted into the vagina on its own to inactivate sperm or be used with other barrier methods like diaphragms and cervical caps. *Which type of condom does not prevent the transmission of STIs and HIV?*

© Planned Parenthood Federation of America

Using an External Condom

Applying an External Condom

1. Gently tear open the condom package at its edge. Do not use teeth or scissors to do this. If the package is wet or sticky, discard it. Each condom is rolled into a ring within its package.
2. Determine which way the condom unrolls using a finger.
3. Pinch the condom tip to remove air. This will prevent breakage when the condom fills with semen. Leave a small amount of space at the tip to collect semen.
4. Place the condom at the tip of the erect penis.
5. The condom will not roll if it is placed incorrectly. Once the condom is positioned correctly, roll it to the base of the penis.
6. Apply some water-based lubricant if the condom is not lubricated. Never use petroleum-based lotions or lubricants such as Vaseline with a latex condom.

Removing an External Condom

1. Remove the penis from the partner's genitals before it softens. Otherwise, the condom can fall off and spill semen.
2. Hold the base of the condom at its ring while withdrawing to keep the condom from coming off the penis.
3. Pull off the condom and dispose of it in the trash. Wash your hands.
4. Never reuse a condom. Use a new condom for each erection.

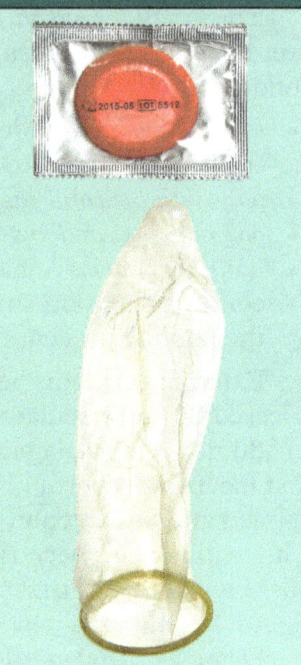

Top to bottom: kaarsten/Shutterstock.com; Dragan Milovanovic/Shutterstock.com

Figure 24.5 To effectively prevent pregnancy, a person must know when and how to apply and remove an external condom. *Why should people not use external condoms past their expiration date?*

Using an Internal Condom

Applying an Internal Condom

1. Apply spermicide to the inside of the inner ring of the condom.
2. Squeeze the inner ring at the closed end of the condom and push it into the vagina as deep as it will go. The outer ring should rest just outside the vagina.
3. Hold the outer ring against the vaginal opening while the penis is inserted. The penis should not slide outside the condom.

Removing an Internal Condom

1. Hold the outer ring and twist the end of the condom to trap semen inside and prevent spillage.
2. Pull the condom out and discard it in the trash. An internal condom can only be used once. A new condom must be used each time a person has sexual intercourse.

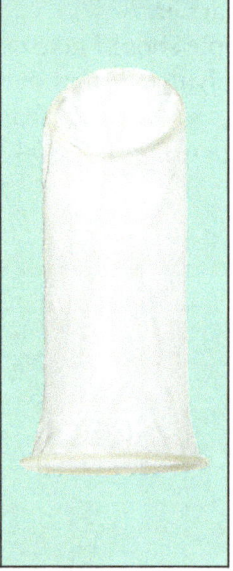

© Planned Parenthood Federation of America

Figure 24.6 People should take care to insert and remove an internal condom properly to prevent semen from spilling. *What can make internal condoms more effective?*

Internal Condoms

An *internal condom*, sometimes called a *female condom*, is a device similar to a pouch, which is placed inside the vagina. Internal condoms are made of plastic, so they do not cause allergic reactions in people allergic to latex. Each end of the condom has a flexible ring to help a person insert the condom and to hold it in place while the penis is inserted. Internal condoms are more effective if a person adds spermicide to the inside or withdraws the penis before ejaculation.

An internal condom must be inserted before the penis touches a partner's genitals. It prevents pregnancy by catching semen. It also forms a barrier to STIs (**Figure 24.6**). An internal condom should not be worn with an external condom, since friction between them reduces effectiveness.

Contraceptive Sponge

The **contraceptive sponge** is a barrier method that helps block sperm from entering the uterus (**Figure 24.7**). The contraceptive sponge is inserted into the vagina and positioned to cover the cervix. A person can insert it several hours (at least 10 minutes) before sexual intercourse and leave it in place for 30 hours.

Unlike condoms, the contraceptive sponge does not have to be replaced each time people have sexual intercourse. The same sponge can be used more than once during a 30-hour period. A small loop makes it easier to pull out of the vagina.

The contraceptive sponge does not protect against STIs and HIV, so the female's partner should still wear a condom. Contraceptive sponges are less effective in preventing pregnancy than external and internal condoms. They are more effective at preventing pregnancy for people who have never given birth, as compared to people who have given birth.

contraceptive sponge contraceptive device made of plastic foam; covers the cervix to prevent sperm from entering the uterus and contains spermicide

Diaphragm

The **diaphragm** is a flexible, cup-shaped disk that is inserted into the vagina. It covers the cervix and helps block sperm from entering the uterus (**Figure 24.8**). Unlike with condoms and contraceptive sponges, getting a diaphragm requires an exam and prescription. During the exam, the healthcare professional checks the health of the cervix and uterus and prescribes the correctly sized diaphragm. A person can then purchase a diaphragm with a prescription at drugstores.

The diaphragm's package contains directions for correct insertion, removal, and care. A person must use it each time intercourse occurs and cover it with spermicide before insertion. Spermicide causes the sperm to stop moving and prevents them from entering the uterus.

diaphragm cup-shaped contraceptive device made of silicone; covers the cervix to prevent sperm from entering the uterus and is bigger than the cervical cap

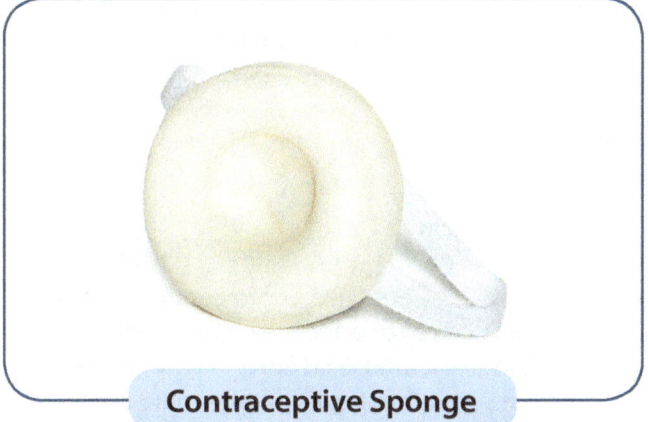

Figure 24.7 A contraceptive sponge is made of plastic foam, is about 2 inches in diameter, and contains spermicide.

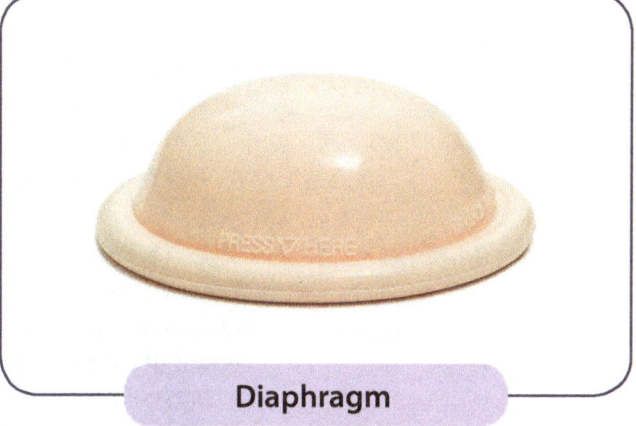

Figure 24.8 Diaphragms are made of silicone, a material that usually does not cause discomfort. *What part of the body does a diaphragm cover?*

cervical cap cup-shaped contraceptive device made of silicone; covers the cervix to prevent sperm from entering the uterus and is smaller than the diaphragm

A diaphragm costs more than a condom or contraceptive sponge, but a person can use it multiple times and for much longer than other barrier methods. While initial costs are relatively high, the diaphragm is inexpensive for long-term contraception.

Cervical Cap

The **cervical cap** is a flexible cup that covers the cervix and helps block sperm from entering the uterus (**Figure 24.9**). Like the diaphragm, the cervical cap is made of silicone. A person must see a doctor or other healthcare professional to obtain a prescription for a cervical cap. During the exam, a doctor checks the health of the cervix and uterus and prescribes the correct size. The cervical cap works best for people who have never given birth.

The cervical cap's package contains directions for correct insertion, removal, and care. A person must cover the cap with spermicide and insert it before intercourse. Like the diaphragm, the cervical cap is expensive at first, but can be used for a long time.

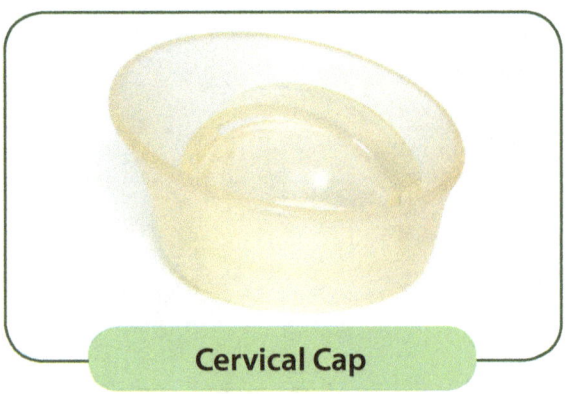

Figure 24.9 The cervical cap is smaller than a diaphragm and may be more difficult to position correctly.

© Planned Parenthood Federation of America

Lesson 24.2 Review

Know and Understand
1. Which barrier methods are worn by females to prevent pregnancy? by males?
2. Which type of condom does *not* also protect against STIs?
3. When during sexual activity should an external or internal condom be applied?
4. What are the similarities and differences between the contraceptive sponge, diaphragm, and cervical cap?

Think Critically
5. What factors might make external and internal condoms difficult to use correctly?
6. Choose two barrier methods and compare them in terms of effectiveness, ease of use, and cost. What factors might affect which method people choose?

REAL WORLD Health Skills

Practice Health-Enhancing Behaviors To be effective, contraceptive methods need to be used correctly every time. On a piece of paper, brainstorm factors that might get in the way of people using barrier methods and abstinence effectively to prevent pregnancy and STIs. Then, list several strategies people could use to make sure they use these methods correctly. Create a journal entry reflecting on what strategies might work best for you now and in the future.

Hormonal Methods

Lesson 24.3

Essential Question: How do hormonal methods work to prevent pregnancy?

Learning Outcomes

After studying this lesson, you will be able to
- understand how hormonal methods prevent pregnancy;
- distinguish between different types of oral contraceptives;
- explain the use of the birth control patch;
- describe the function of the vaginal ring;
- identify what a person must do to get the birth control shot;
- analyze the effectiveness of the birth control implant;
- contrast the two types of intrauterine devices (IUDs); and
- explain how emergency contraception helps prevent pregnancy after sexual intercourse.

Key Terms

birth control implant
birth control patch
birth control shot
emergency contraception
intrauterine device (IUD)
oral contraceptives
vaginal ring

Warm-Up Activity

What Are the Facts?

Access Information What do you already know about hormonal contraceptive methods? For each hormonal method listed, indicate whether you have never heard of it, have heard of it, or know how it works. Share what you know with a partner and then use a reliable resource to verify two facts you and your partner think you know. Were your facts correct? Verify the other facts you shared as you read this lesson.

Method	Never Heard of It	Heard of It	Know How It Works
Birth control implant			
Birth control patch			
Birth control pill			
Birth control shot			
Emergency contraceptive pill			
Intrauterine device (IUD)			
Vaginal ring			

Hormonal methods of contraception prevent pregnancy by using *hormones*, or chemical substances that control many body functions, including reproduction. Hormonal methods of contraception use the hormones estrogen and *progestin* (synthetic progesterone) to thicken cervical mucus, thin the endometrial lining of the uterus, and inhibit *ovulation*, which is the release of an egg. Because hormonal methods work in this way, they also help control the menstrual cycle to treat severe menstrual pain, endometriosis, and other reproductive disorders.

		Hormonal Methods		
Method	Use	Requires a Doctor's Visit	Estimated Cost	Number of Pregnancies Expected (per 100 Females)
Birth control implant	A small rod implanted into the body by a doctor; releases hormones to prevent ovulation and must be replaced after five years	Yes	$0–$1,300 (including doctor's visit), depending on insurance	Fewer than 1
Intrauterine device (IUD)	A device inserted into the uterus by a doctor; repels sperm; hormonal IUDs also release hormones to thicken cervical mucus and inhibit ovulation; is effective for 3–12 years	Yes	$0–$1,300 (including doctor's visit), depending on insurance	Fewer than 1
Birth control shot	An injection of hormones by a doctor every three months; prevents ovulation	Yes	$0–$250 (including doctor's visit), depending on insurance	6
Birth control patch	A patch placed on the skin every week for three weeks; releases hormones to prevent ovulation	Yes	$0–$150 per month, depending on insurance	9
Birth control pill	A pill taken every day; contains hormones that prevent ovulation	Yes	$0–$50 per month, depending on insurance	9
Vaginal ring	A flexible ring inserted into the vagina; releases hormones to prevent ovulation and must be replaced monthly	Yes	$0–$200 per month, depending on insurance	9
Emergency contraceptive pill	A pill taken within five days of sexual intercourse; contains hormones that prevent ovulation	Yes (ella®); No (Plan B One-Step®)	$50–$67 (ella®); $40–$50 (Plan B One-Step®)	15 (ella®); 11–25 (Plan B One-Step®)

Figure 24.10 Most hormonal methods require a doctor's visit, but each type will vary in cost, effectiveness, and how long it will last. *Which two hormones are used in hormonal methods of contraception?*

In this lesson, you will learn about several types of hormonal methods (**Figure 24.10**). All of these methods use hormones to influence the female reproductive system. No hormonal methods currently exist for males, but several different options are being researched and developed.

Oral Contraceptives

Oral contraceptives are medications containing hormones that reduce the likelihood of pregnancy. These medications are taken *orally* (by mouth) at the same time each day (**Figure 24.11**). The hormones in birth control pills help prevent pregnancy by preventing ovulation, or the release of an egg, and thickening cervical mucus to slow sperm down. If ovulation does not occur, there is no egg for a sperm to fertilize. Birth control pills do not prevent STIs or HIV. In fact, some research suggests people who use birth control pills have an increased risk of STIs.

People need to visit a doctor or other healthcare professional and get a prescription to begin taking birth control pills. During the exam, a doctor will make sure no health conditions will make taking the pill dangerous. The pill is very effective at preventing pregnancy if taken *exactly as prescribed*. Skipping even one pill increases the chance of becoming pregnant.

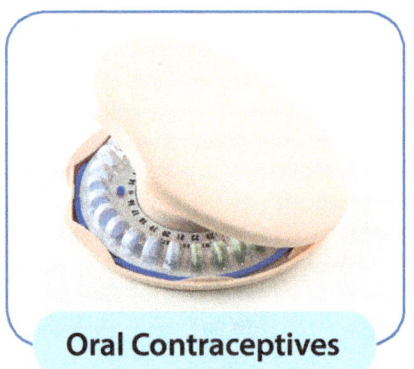

Oral Contraceptives

Jacob Kearns/Shutterstock.com

Figure 24.11 Oral contraceptives are usually called the *birth control pill* or just *the pill*.

oral contraceptives medications containing hormones that stop ovulation; are taken every day

Local and Global Health

The Impact of the Pill

The birth control pill, introduced in 1960, was a breakthrough in contraception. In the US today, about 16 percent of females ages 15–49 take the birth control pill. Around the world, this number is closer to 9 percent.

When it was introduced, the pill gave females an effective way to plan and space pregnancies. This and other factors contributed to social change. Since 1960, the number of females in the workplace has tripled, and females have more financial independence. Before 1960, only 6 percent of females in the US completed a college education. This number rose to 37 percent in the decades after.

Apart from contraception, the birth control pill also has other health benefits. Taking the birth control pill reduces menstrual cramping, symptoms of endometriosis, premenstrual syndrome (PMS), and the risks of an ectopic pregnancy and ovarian and uterine cancer. Females have lighter periods using the pill, which helps prevent iron deficiency and anemia.

The birth control pill has also benefited females globally, though some countries have not seen as much social change. Fewer females with low incomes bear the economic burden of raising more children, and fewer females fear the health risks of pregnancy and childbirth.

 Practice Your Skills

Access Information

Since the birth control pill was introduced, it has evolved and become a safer and more reliable method of contraception. In a small group, use reliable resources to research answers to the following questions about the birth control pill and its evolution:

- What were the first birth control pills like? How have these pills changed over the years?
- What are the potential side effects of taking birth control pills? Have these effects changed over time? What precautions help protect females from these side effects?
- How exactly do birth control pills prevent pregnancy? How effective are they?
- Where can females go to learn more about or get birth control pills?

Many people use apps or alarms to help them remember to take the pill (**Figure 24.12**). The birth control pill comes in two basic forms: the combination pill and the progestin-only pill.

Combination Pill

Most people who take birth control pills take the *combination pill*, which contains the hormones estrogen and progestin. The combination pill comes in a pack of 21, 28, 91, or 365 pills. All of these packs have *active pills*, which contain hormones. Packs of 28 and 91 also have *inactive pills*, which do not contain hormones and help a person stay in the habit of taking a pill every day. Packs of 91 or 365 pills are sometimes called *continuous* or *extended-cycle birth control*. Following is a summary of these options:

- **21-pill pack:** Someone using the 21-pill pack takes an active pill every day for three weeks and then no pills for one week. After that week, the person starts a new 21-pill pack.

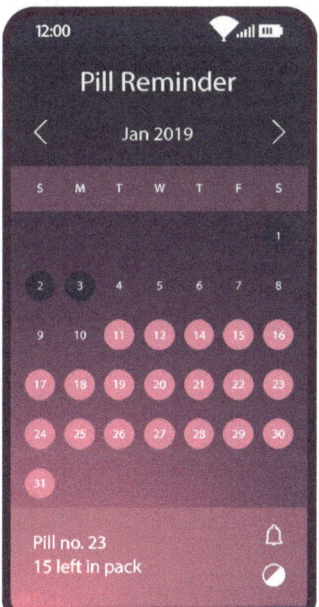

Some apps can
- send reminders to take the pill
- provide advice if you skip a pill
- track symptoms to spot any side effects of the pill
- record and analyze how your menstrual cycle changes over time
- predict when you will begin menstruating or ovulating

bsd/Shutterstock.com

Figure 24.12 Any information an app provides about a female's menstrual cycle should come from a reliable source.

- **28-pill pack:** Someone using the 28-pill pack takes one active pill each day for three weeks, then one inactive pill every day for one week. The last seven pills have no effect on the female reproductive system, but help with keeping the daily habit of taking the pill.
- **91-pill pack:** Someone using the 91-pill pack takes active pills for 12 weeks and inactive pills for one week.
- **365-pill pack:** These packs contain 365 active pills that are taken each day.

When using packs of 21, 28, or 91 pills, females experience *withdrawal bleeding* while taking the inactive pills. This bleeding is not the same as menstruation (the shedding of the uterus's thickened lining). Active pills make the uterine lining shed during withdrawal bleeding much thinner.

Progestin-Only Pill

Some people take a form of the birth control pill that contains only progestin. This *progestin-only pill*, also called the *minipill*, contains no estrogen. The progestin-only pill comes in a 28-pill pack, and all of the pills contain active hormones. People who take the progestin-only pill tend to experience fewer side effects.

birth control patch plastic contraceptive device applied to the skin as a patch; releases hormones to stop ovulation

Birth Control Patch

The **birth control patch** (often called the *patch*) is a thin, 2- to 3-inch, plastic patch applied to the skin like a bandage (**Figure 24.13**). The patch works like the birth control pill, except that hormones are absorbed in a *transdermal* way (from the patch through the skin into the blood). The birth control patch prevents ovulation and thickens cervical mucus, slowing down sperm.

Females who use this method apply one patch to the skin for one week and then remove it. They replace the old patch with a new patch for the second week. After removing the second patch, they wear a third patch for the third week. No patch is worn during the fourth week (during withdrawal bleeding).

The patch's package contains directions for applying and removing birth control patches. The patch must be worn in specific locations. The directions should state what people should do if a patch falls off or they forget to replace one.

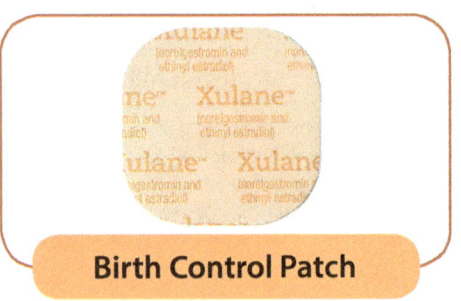

Birth Control Patch

© Planned Parenthood Federation of America

Figure 24.13 Like the birth control pill, the patch contains the hormones estrogen and progestin.

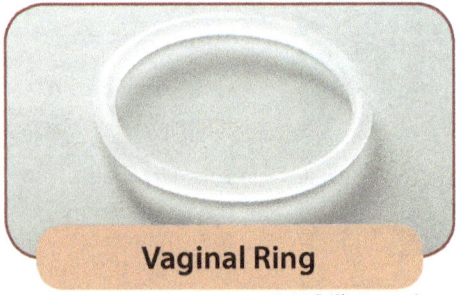

Vaginal Ring

Image Point Fr/Shutterstock.com

Figure 24.14 People should follow the package's directions for proper storage, insertion, and removal of the vaginal ring. *For how long is a vaginal ring used?*

vaginal ring flexible, ring-shaped contraceptive device inserted into the vagina; releases hormones to stop ovulation

Vaginal Ring

The **vaginal ring** is a small, flexible ring that contains the hormones estrogen and progestin (**Figure 24.14**). The ring works by releasing hormones that prevent ovulation and thicken cervical mucus to slow sperm movement.

The vaginal ring is inserted into the vagina for three consecutive weeks. Exactly three weeks after insertion, a person should remove the ring, ideally at the same time it was inserted, and discard it. No ring is used during the fourth week (during withdrawal bleeding).

Birth Control Shot

The **birth control shot**, often called *Depo-Provera*, is an injection of the hormone progestin. The progestin in the shot helps prevent pregnancy by preventing ovulation and thickening cervical mucus. A female who uses this method must see a healthcare professional to receive the shot every three months. Depending on the type of shot, it can be given in the arm or buttocks. The birth control shot is highly effective in preventing pregnancy if a person receives injections according to schedule.

Birth Control Implant

The **birth control implant** is a flexible, toothpick-sized rod containing the hormone progestin (**Figure 24.15**). The implant releases progestin, which prevents ovulation and thickens cervical mucus. The implant can be left in place for three or four years, during which time it gradually releases doses of progestin.

Intrauterine Device (IUD)

An **intrauterine device (IUD)** is a small, T-shaped device a doctor inserts into the uterus. IUDs can also be removed by a doctor, making IUDs a reversible method of contraception. Two types of IUDs exist: copper IUDs (*ParaGard®*) and hormonal IUDs (*Mirena®, Liletta®, Skyla®,* or *Kyleena®*) (**Figure 24.16**). These IUDs work in different ways to prevent pregnancy:

- **Copper IUD:** The copper ParaGard® IUD is thought to interfere with sperm movement, fertilization, and implantation. The advantage of the ParaGard® IUD is it can be left in place for 12 years and does not affect a person's hormone levels. The ParaGard® IUD can also be used as a form of emergency contraception.
- **Hormonal IUDs:** Hormonal IUDs release hormones that inhibit ovulation and cause mucus in the cervix to thicken, making it difficult for sperm to reach the uterus. Hormonal IUDs last for years and can reduce menstrual cramps and significantly lighten or even stop menstruation.

Both copper and hormonal IUDs can be removed if a female wants to become pregnant.

birth control shot contraceptive method in which a female receives an injection of progestin every three months to stop ovulation

birth control implant flexible, toothpick-sized contraceptive device inserted under the skin of the upper arm; releases progestin to stop ovulation

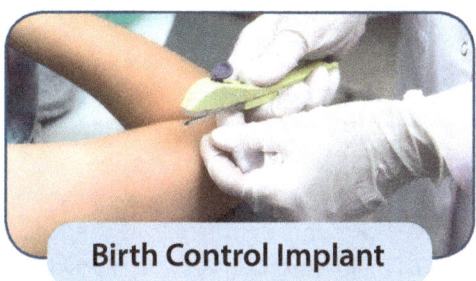

Birth Control Implant

PAKULA PIOTR/Shutterstock.com

Figure 24.15 A doctor inserts the birth control implant under the skin of a female's upper arm, where the implant releases progestin.

intrauterine device (IUD) small, T-shaped contraceptive device inserted into the uterus; copper IUDs interfere with sperm movement, and hormonal IUDs release hormones to thicken cervical mucus and inhibit ovulation

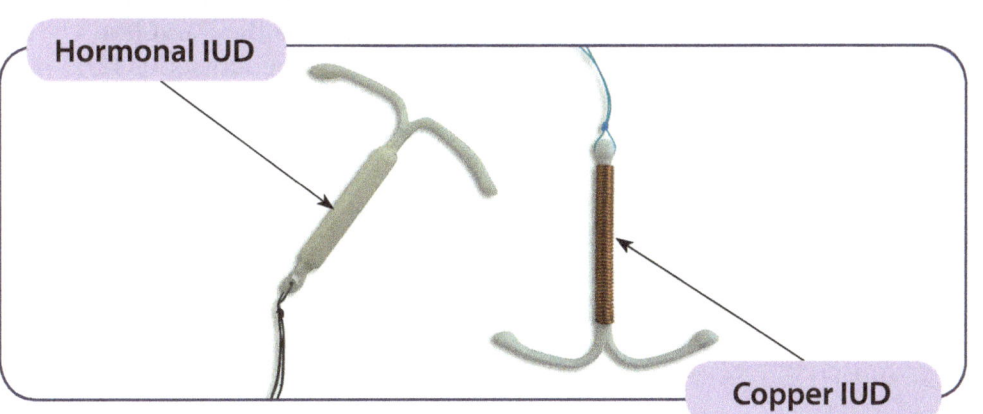

iStock.com/Lalocracio

Figure 24.16 Both copper and hormonal IUDs must be inserted and removed by a doctor. *Into what female reproductive organ is an IUD inserted?*

Research in Action

Hormonal Contraceptives for Males

Since the introduction of the birth control pill, females have had access to long-term, reversible hormonal contraception. These contraceptive methods include oral contraceptives; the birth control shot, patch, or implant; the vaginal ring; and IUDs. Each method reduces the risk of pregnancy.

In recent years, scientists have also been testing the safety and effectiveness of hormonal contraceptives for males. Two oral contraceptives have been tested in small groups of males. One is called *dimethandrolone undecanoate*, and the other is called *11-beta-MNTDC*. Both oral contraceptives contain a combination of hormones that lower testosterone production in males. Since testosterone is needed for sperm production, a drop in testosterone means the testes stop making sperm. These oral contraceptives are taken once daily and affect sperm production after two to three months. Sperm production begins again a few days after a male stops taking the pills.

 Practice Your Skills

Comprehend Concepts

With a partner, discuss why it is important to have hormonal contraceptive methods available for both males and females. What advantages would hormonal contraceptives have over other forms of contraception for males? During your discussion, complete the table that follows comparing the advantages and disadvantages of different methods of male contraception. Research any method with which you are not familiar. If a male hormonal contraceptive was approved, do you think males would use it? Why or why not?

Male Contraceptive Methods	Advantages	Disadvantages
Sexual abstinence		
External condom		
Sterilization		
Withdrawal		
Male hormonal contraceptive pill		

Emergency Contraception

Even when partners agree to use contraception and try to use it correctly, mistakes can happen. For example, an external condom can break, leak, or slip off. An internal condom might leak or slip out of position. A person might forget to insert a diaphragm or take the birth control pill.

In these cases, **emergency contraception** can help prevent pregnancy. Emergency contraception can also help prevent pregnancy in the case of sexual assault. One type of emergency contraception is the ParaGard® copper IUD. If inserted within five days of sexual intercourse, this IUD is the most effective method of emergency contraception.

Several types of emergency contraceptive pills can also prevent pregnancy. These pills, such as *ella®* and *Plan B One-Step®*, contain hormones that prevent ovulation and thicken cervical mucus. Emergency contraception is similar to other hormonal methods, but contains a greater amount of the same hormones. Emergency contraception prevents fertilization. It does *not* stop or interrupt a pregnancy that has already occurred. It also does not reduce the risk of STIs and HIV.

emergency contraception contraceptive method used to prevent pregnancy when normal contraception has failed; includes the copper ParaGard® IUD and emergency contraceptive pills containing hormones

Most emergency contraceptive pills are available at drugstores without a prescription, and anyone can buy them, regardless of age. The emergency contraceptive pill ella® requires a doctor's prescription and is the most effective emergency contraceptive pill. Emergency contraceptive pills can reduce the chance of pregnancy by up to 89 percent when used within five days of sexual intercourse. The earlier emergency contraception is taken, the more effective it will be.

While effective as a backup method, emergency contraception is less effective than standard birth control pills and several other contraceptive methods. Emergency contraception is not intended for regular use and should not be used as regular birth control for several reasons. Long-term use can cause irregular and unpredictable menstruation. Other forms of contraception are much less expensive and much more effective.

Lesson 24.3 Review

Know and Understand
1. What hormones are used in hormonal contraceptives to inhibit ovulation in females?
2. Explain the difference between active and inactive pills in oral contraceptives.
3. How is the vaginal ring different from the diaphragm or cervical cap?
4. Describe the difference between the birth control patch, shot, and implant.
5. Which type of IUD does not affect a female's hormone levels?

Think Critically
6. What factors do you think influence whether a female chooses to take oral contraceptives or use another hormonal method?
7. How is emergency contraception different from other hormonal methods of contraception? How is it different from the decision to end a pregnancy?

✓ REAL WORLD Health Skills

Communicate with Others As a class, identify a person in your community who is an expert on hormonal contraceptives. This person could be a gynecologist, doctor, or therapist or counselor who specializes in sexual health. As a class, schedule an interview with this person or contact the person electronically to ask about hormonal contraceptive options. Get answers to the following questions about each hormonal contraceptive method:
- How effective is this method, and what factors influence effectiveness?
- What are the short-term side effects?
- What are the long-term side effects?
- Are teens more likely to have side effects compared to adults?
- How much does it cost?
- What are the advantages and disadvantages of using this method?
- How old do you have to be to purchase this contraceptive?

Lesson 24.4

Natural Methods and Sterilization

Essential Question
How do natural methods and sterilization help reduce the risk of pregnancy?

Key Terms
fertility awareness method (FAM)
tubal ligation
vasectomy
withdrawal

Learning Outcomes

After studying this lesson, you will be able to

- explain how fertility awareness methods (FAM) reduce the risk of pregnancy;
- analyze why the withdrawal method is ineffective;
- describe the process of male sterilization; and
- explain how female sterilization is performed.

Warm-Up Activity

Thoughts and Decisions

Analyze Influences Read the statements that follow and write what thoughts come to mind when you read each one. Have you ever thought something similar to these statements? How have these thoughts influenced your decisions? As you read this lesson, refer back to these statements and note how your thoughts about them change. How might your thoughts about them influence your decisions in the future?

- I know my body. We won't get pregnant if we have sex today.
- I've been watching the calendar for a month. I can't get pregnant, so there's no need for a condom.
- If I just withdraw, nothing will get inside.

In this lesson, you will learn about natural methods of contraception and sterilization. Natural methods are methods that do not use barriers, devices, or hormones. Instead, these methods prevent pregnancy by tracking a female's cycle of fertility and taking actions such as withdrawal during sexual intercourse. Sterilization involves physically altering the reproductive system, usually permanently (**Figure 24.17**).

Natural Methods

Some people prefer natural methods of contraception because they do not use devices or medications. This preference might be a result of a person's values and beliefs or medical reasons. Additionally, the cost of contraceptive devices or medications may mean some people want to use natural methods, which do not cost money. Although they are less expensive, natural methods are harder to use correctly, which means they are less effective at preventing pregnancy for most people.

Natural Methods and Sterilization

Method	Use	Requires a Doctor's Visit	Estimated Cost	Number of Pregnancies Expected (per 100 Females)
Tubal ligation (female sterilization)	Surgery to cut or block the fallopian tubes	Yes	$0–$6,000 (including doctor's visit), depending on insurance	Fewer than 1
Vasectomy (male sterilization)	Surgery to cut or block the vas deferens, which transport sperm from the testes to the penis	Yes	$0–$1,000 (including doctor's visit), depending on insurance	Fewer than 1
Fertility awareness methods (FAM)	Methods that track a female's fertile (unsafe) and infertile (safe) days; include the temperature method, cervical mucus method, and calendar method	No (but recommended)	$0–$20	12–24
Withdrawal	Pulling the penis out of the vagina before ejaculation	No	$0	22

Figure 24.17 Natural methods do not require a doctor's visit and are usually free. Sterilization can be expensive, depending on insurance, and requires a doctor's visit. *How many pregnancies are expected when using tubal ligation?*

Fertility Awareness Methods (FAM)

A **fertility awareness method (FAM)** is a contraceptive method that takes advantage of the natural rhythm of a female's fertility. People who use FAM track when ovulation occurs and which days an egg is capable of being fertilized. As you know, the menstrual cycle typically lasts 28 days. In general, sexual intercourse on seven of those days can result in an egg being fertilized. This is because an egg lives for about one day, while sperm can live for three to five days. This means pregnancy is possible three to five days before ovulation, on the day of ovulation, and on the first and possibly second day after ovulation.

FAM is extremely useful for planning a pregnancy, but is only somewhat helpful for preventing pregnancy. There are several types of FAM:

- **Temperature method:** A person can track ovulation by measuring *basal body temperature* (resting temperature) first thing every morning. Body temperature rises slightly after ovulation and stays higher than normal for most of the remainder of that menstrual cycle. Temperature drops back to normal near the end of the cycle, when menstruation begins. To prevent pregnancy, someone should only have sex three days after body temperature rises until temperature declines (about the time of menstruation). During ovulation, body temperature rises just tenths of a degree. Because the change is so small, people should use a special basal temperature thermometer and record daily temperatures on a chart or app.

fertility awareness method (FAM) contraceptive method that tracks a female's cycle of fertility and avoids sexual activity on days an egg can be fertilized

A female's body temperature might change at any time due to alcohol consumption, sleep, stress, or other factors. For this reason, people should record several months of temperature readings so they can recognize natural variations.

- **Cervical mucus method:** *Mucus* is a thick, watery secretion present in many parts of the body, including the cervix. The consistency of cervical mucus changes during the menstrual cycle (**Figure 24.18**). According to this method, pregnancy can occur two or three days before slippery mucus begins, for about three days after slippery mucus reaches its greatest amount, and possibly at the end of menstruation. Pregnancy is less likely when slippery mucus begins to decline, when mucus becomes sticky or cloudy, and during the dry days that follow this decline. Females examine cervical mucus by placing their fingers inside their vagina or examining mucus discharged on their underwear. Many extraneous factors can affect a female's cervical mucus.

- **Calendar-based methods:** People using a calendar-based method mark the day a female begins menstruating and then mark days pregnancy is likely or unlikely to occur. Generally, pregnancy will not occur during the six days following the beginning of menstruation and during days 19–32 after menstruation begins. People may use calendars, apps, or cycle beads to keep track of days. Calendar-based methods are not precise. A female's cycle can change at any time due to illness or stress. This method is especially unreliable for people with irregular cycles.

FAM has several drawbacks. FAM requires attention and record keeping and is subject to many mistakes. This is why many people use several methods of FAM together. Still, many people who use FAM do not use the methods regularly and correctly. As a result, about 25 out of 100 people become pregnant, which is a very high rate of pregnancy compared to other contraceptive methods. Furthermore, FAM does not prevent STIs. FAM is best for people who are in a position to raise and support a child. For these reasons, FAM is not recommended for teens.

Figure 24.18 A female can determine likelihood of a pregnancy occurring based on the consistency of cervical mucus.

Cervical Mucus During the Menstrual Cycle

Stage	Cervical Mucus
Menstruation	Blood flow prevents observation of mucus.
Post-menstruation	Little or no mucus is present (*dry days*).
Pre-ovulation	Mucus increases and is yellow or cloudy and sticky. Just before ovulation, mucus becomes clear and slippery for four days (*slippery days*).
Ovulation	Mucus is very wet, thick, and sticky.
Post-ovulation	Mucus reduces and becomes cloudy.
Pre-menstruation	Little or no mucus is present, especially one to two days before menstruation.

Withdrawal

Withdrawal, or *pulling out*, is one of the least effective contraceptive methods. When people use withdrawal, a male pulls the penis out of the female's vagina before ejaculating. This may keep sperm out of the vagina and reduce the risk of pregnancy.

Withdrawal is *not* an effective method of preventing pregnancy for several reasons. Withdrawal is difficult to time correctly and requires self-control. It is not always easy for a male to withdraw during intense sexual excitement. In addition, before ejaculation, *pre-ejaculate fluid* containing sperm can leak from the penis and cause pregnancy. Withdrawal results in many pregnancies and does not protect people from STIs (**Figure 24.19**).

withdrawal contraceptive method that involves pulling the penis out of the vagina before ejaculation

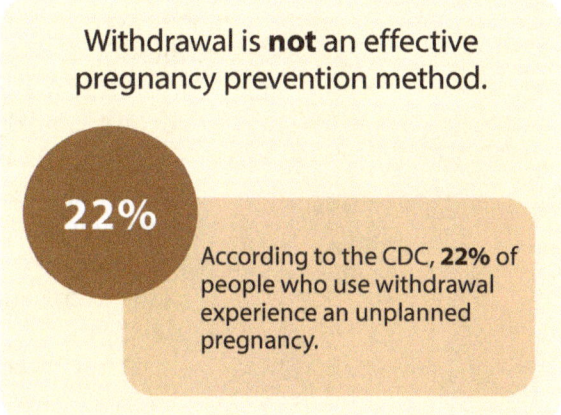

Figure 24.19 When used alone, withdrawal is one of the most ineffective methods of contraception. *How can a person become pregnant even if a penis is withdrawn before ejaculation?*

Sterilization

Sterilization prevents pregnancy by permanently altering the male or female reproductive system. These alterations work by preventing the sperm and egg from uniting. They do not protect against STIs and HIV.

Sterilization may be the best choice for adults who know they do not want children or any more children. Sterilization is not appropriate for everyone, however. Reversing sterilization is difficult and often unsuccessful. Therefore, people considering sterilization must be sure they do not ever want children (**Figure 24.20**).

Choosing Sterilization	
Reasons to Choose Sterilization	**Reasons Not to Choose Sterilization**
• Adults know they do not want to have more children. • Adults find other contraceptive methods unacceptable. Hormonal methods may be dangerous for some people, or pregnancy may carry serious risks. • Adults have a genetic disease or disorder they do not want to pass on to children. • Adults know they are and will never be emotionally or financially able to raise a family.	• Adults might want children, but do not want them now. If there is *any* chance adults might someday want children, they should not select sterilization. • Adults feel pressured to be sterilized. Adults should make their own decisions since they will live with the effects. • Adults have other personal issues, such as financial or personal stress or relationship conflict. These problems might go away; sterilization will not.

Figure 24.20 There are many reasons to choose sterilization, but adults should be aware that sterilization is often irreversible.

Male Sterilization

vasectomy surgical procedure that cuts or blocks the vas deferens, permanently preventing pregnancy

Male sterilization involves a surgery called a **vasectomy**, which a doctor performs. During a vasectomy, the *vas deferens* (two tubes that carry sperm from the testes to the penis) are cut or blocked. This prevents sperm from leaving the testes and entering semen. Vasectomy is nearly 100 percent effective.

A doctor usually performs a vasectomy in a doctor's office or hospital. The surgery involves making a small incision or puncture in each side of the scrotum. The doctor then cuts or blocks the vas deferens through this incision (**Figure 24.21**).

Most males who have a vasectomy return home the same day and recover quickly with no side effects. Some males experience bruising, swelling, and discomfort after the procedure. After a vasectomy, the prostate and seminal vesicles continue to function. Males still ejaculate normally and continue to produce semen. The testes keep making testosterone, so males can get erections and have sex just as they did prior to the surgery. Vasectomies are much less expensive than female sterilization.

After three months, a doctor will use an X-ray to confirm the vas deferens were successfully blocked. People should use an alternative form of contraception until that time.

Female Sterilization

Female sterilization works by blocking the fallopian tubes, which prevents sperm from reaching an egg released from an ovary. It does not affect the function of the ovaries. A female continues to make female hormones and ovulate after this procedure. Sterilization does not affect a female's sexual characteristics, sexual arousal, ability to have sex, or onset of menopause.

tubal ligation surgical procedure that cuts or blocks the fallopian tubes, permanently preventing pregnancy

The surgical procedure for female sterilization is **tubal ligation** (**Figure 24.22**). This surgery makes it impossible for sperm to reach an egg, which means that tubal ligation is nearly 100 percent effective in preventing pregnancy.

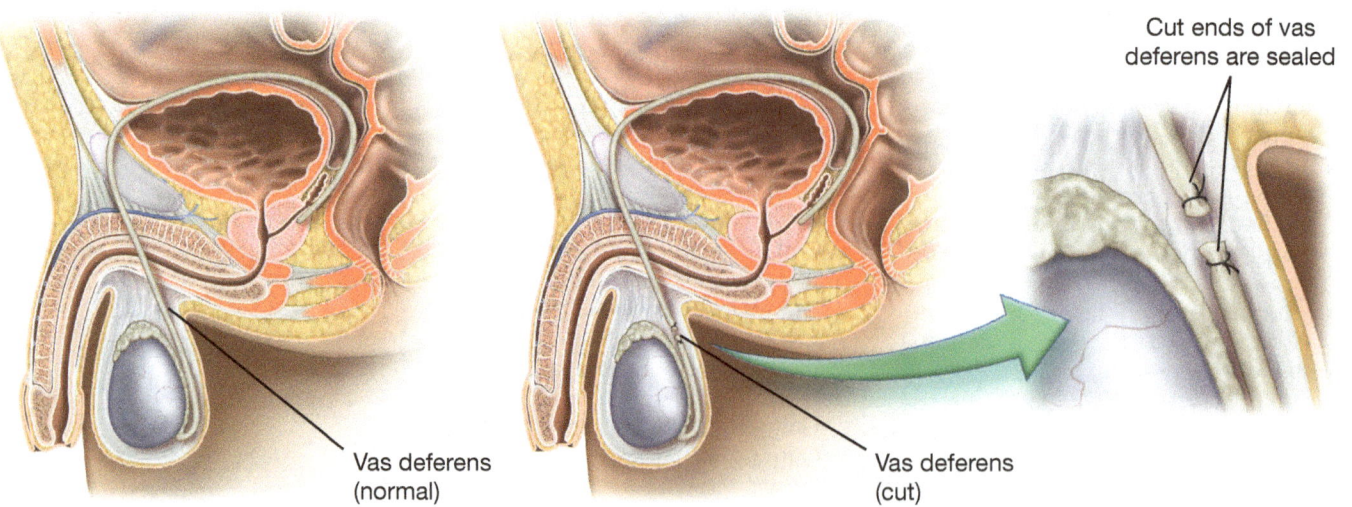

© Body Scientific International

Figure 24.21 In a vasectomy, the vas deferens are cut or blocked and then sealed to stop the release of sperm.

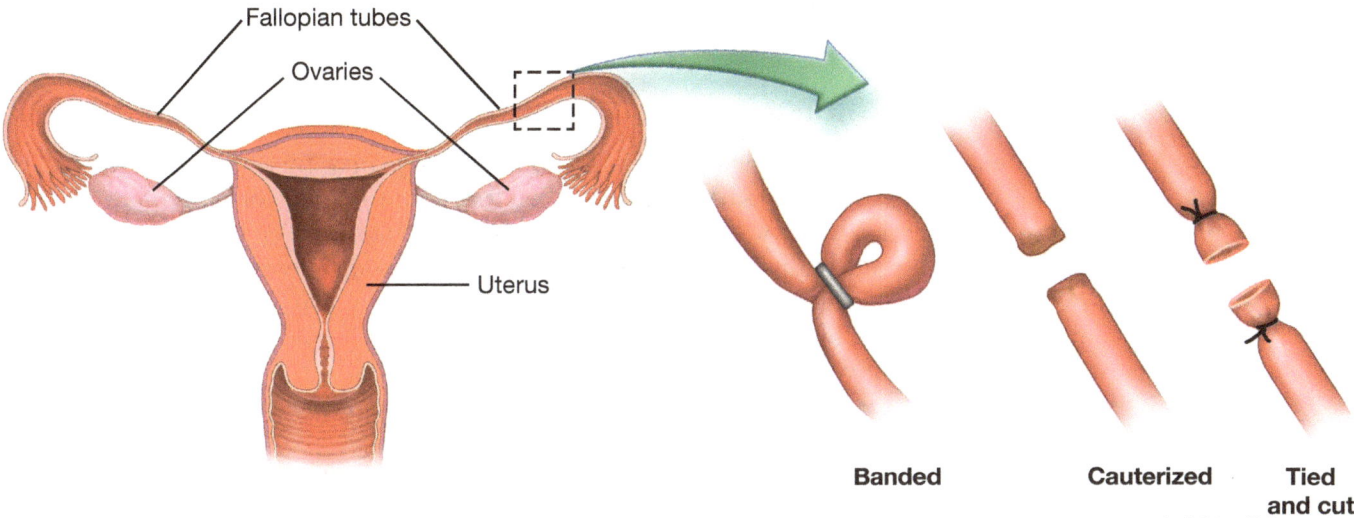

Figure 24.22 In tubal ligation, a doctor cuts or blocks the fallopian tubes. *How does tubal ligation affect the function of the ovaries?*

Many tubal ligations are done in a hospital, while others are done in an outpatient surgery clinic. Depending on the type of surgery, some females return home the same day, while others recover in the hospital. Three months after surgery, doctors view an X-ray to confirm the tubes were successfully blocked. During those first three months, people should use an alternative form of contraception.

Lesson 24.4 Review

Know and Understand
1. Why is FAM not recommended for teens?
2. Explain why withdrawal is not an effective method of contraception.
3. Why should people be sure they never want children before choosing sterilization?

Think Critically
4. What factors make it difficult to track a female's cycle of fertility?
5. What are the similarities and differences between a vasectomy and tubal ligation?

✓ REAL WORLD Health Skills

Analyze Influences With a partner, discuss why people might choose natural methods of contraception over other methods. Why are these methods described as *natural*? What beliefs, ideas, and viewpoints might influence people to prefer these methods? Brainstorm with your partner to analyze these influences. Then, write a paragraph about situations that are appropriate for using natural methods. Create a podcast where you discuss the following question with your partner: *What factors affect people's decisions about contraception? How do these factors change over time?*

Chapter 24 Review and Assessment

Chapter Summary

Contraception includes methods meant to prevent pregnancy. These methods help people plan pregnancy and remain childless when they choose. Having reliable information about contraception is important. Unreliable information can result in an unplanned pregnancy. There are five major types of contraception: sexual abstinence, barrier methods, hormonal methods, natural methods, and sterilization. Emergency contraception can help prevent pregnancy if these methods fail.

The most effective method of contraception is sexual abstinence. Abstinence is also the most effective method of preventing STI and HIV transmission. It has many social and emotional benefits and costs less than other methods.

Barrier methods work by physically blocking sperm from traveling through the female reproductive system and fertilizing an egg. Internal and external condoms are examples of barrier methods that also reduce the risk of STI and HIV transmission. Other barrier methods include the contraceptive sponge, diaphragm, and cervical cap.

Hormonal methods contain hormones that influence the female reproductive system. These methods help prevent pregnancy by thickening cervical mucus, thinning the lining of the uterus, and inhibiting ovulation (the release of an egg). Oral contraceptives are hormone-containing pills a female takes every day. Other methods include the birth control patch, vaginal ring, birth control shot, birth control implant, and intrauterine devices (IUDs). Emergency contraception is a hormonal method that helps prevent pregnancy within five days of sexual intercourse. It does not end a pregnancy that has already begun.

Natural methods of contraception include fertility awareness methods (FAM) and withdrawal. FAM tracks a female's menstrual cycle to time sexual intercourse when there is no egg for sperm to fertilize. Withdrawal involves pulling the penis out of the vagina before ejaculation and is not effective when used alone. Sterilization is a permanent method of birth control that involves surgically altering the reproductive system.

Vocabulary Activity

Write a short dialogue that narrates a discussion between two people about sexual health decisions. In your dialogue, the two people might talk about choosing abstinence or about factors that affect the decision to use a certain type of contraception. They should use effective communication and negotiation skills. Use and define at least five terms from this chapter in your dialogue.

barrier methods	diaphragm	oral contraceptives
birth control implant	emergency contraception	spermicide
birth control patch	fertility awareness method (FAM)	sterilization
birth control shot		tubal ligation
cervical cap	hormonal methods	vaginal ring
contraception	intrauterine device (IUD)	vasectomy
contraceptive sponge	natural methods	withdrawal

Review and Recall

Review the information in this chapter by answering the following questions.

1. Is it possible for someone to become pregnant while menstruating? Explain.
2. Which type of contraception permanently alters the reproductive system?

3. Which contraceptive method protects against STIs and HIV?
   A. condom
   B. birth control pills
   C. sterilization
   D. withdrawal
4. How is emergency contraception different from other forms of contraception?
5. What factors should people consider when choosing a method of contraception?
6. Which method of contraception is most effective at preventing pregnancy and STIs?
7. How do barrier methods work to prevent pregnancy?
8. Explain why a condom should be applied before the penis touches a partner's genitals.
9. Why should an external and internal condom not be worn together?
10. Which of the following does *not* protect against STIs?
    A. sexual abstinence
    B. spermicide
    C. external condom
    D. internal condom
11. Explain how the hormones in birth control pills help prevent pregnancy.
12. Which hormonal method delivers hormones into the blood in a transdermal way?
    A. birth control implant
    B. IUD
    C. birth control patch
    D. birth control implant
13. How often should the birth control shot be given to prevent pregnancy?
14. How does the copper IUD help prevent pregnancy?
15. What are the different forms of emergency contraception?
16. List two factors, besides ovulation, that can change a female's resting body temperature.
17. Which contraceptive method is also called "pulling out"?
18. What are the two surgeries used for male and female sterilization?
19. How long should people use an alternative form of contraception after sterilization?

Standardized Test Prep

Math Practice

Incorrect or inconsistent use decreases the effectiveness of contraception. Read the information below and then answer the following questions.

Effectiveness Rates of Contraception, By Method

Contraceptive Method	Perfect Use	Typical Use
Contraceptive pill	99%	91%
Vaginal ring	99%	91%
Diaphragm	94%	88%
Contraceptive sponge	80–91%	76–88%
External condom	98%	85%
Internal condom	95%	79%
Withdrawal	96%	78%
Spermicide	82%	72%

20. If 5,000 high school students use withdrawal as their primary method of contraception this year, how many will experience a pregnancy?
21. For typical use, what percentage of teens using external condoms will experience a pregnancy?
22. How much more effective is the contraceptive pill than spermicide for perfect use? for typical use?

Chapter 24 Skills Assessment

Critical Thinking Skills
Answer the following questions to assess your knowledge of what you learned in this chapter.

1. What sources of information about sexual health have you accessed? Were these sources reliable? Why or why not?
2. How do people's goals, sexual histories, and any STIs affect decisions about contraception? Explain.
3. What benefits does sexual abstinence have over other forms of contraception? What, if any, weaknesses does it have compared to other forms of contraception?
4. Which barrier methods do you think would be easiest to use? hardest to use? Why?
5. Correct use is an essential part of effectively using barrier methods. Where could you go to get more reliable information about using barrier methods effectively? How would you know the information is reliable?
6. What factors do you think explain why some barrier methods require a doctor's prescription, while others do not?
7. Why do almost all forms of hormonal contraception require a doctor's visit? How does this protect the health of people who use these methods?
8. What resources can people use to learn more about hormonal methods and use them effectively? What apps are available? How do these help with correct use?
9. Which hormonal method do you think would be easiest for someone to use? Why? Explain your reasoning.
10. Do you think most teens understand how emergency contraception works? What misconceptions might teens have? Correct these misconceptions and share with a partner.
11. Why do you think some people prefer natural methods of contraception?
12. Why do many people who use FAM use it to plan a pregnancy and become pregnant?
13. Using reliable resources, research your state's laws about minors' rights to consent to contraceptive services, including sterilization. Discuss these laws in a small group.

Health and Wellness Skills
Complete the following activities to assess your skills related to health and wellness.

14. **Analyze Influences.** Cultural background and beliefs have a significant influence on people's attitudes about teen sexual activity. Consider what beliefs and cultural expectations have shaped your attitude toward teen sexual activity. To do this, you might need to research the different cultures and beliefs in your family. Make a video about your findings and reflect on how these attitudes have influenced your personal opinions about teen sexual activity.
15. **Access Information.** Using reliable resources, research the sterilization options available for males and females. For each sterilization procedure, list what the procedure does, how and where the procedure is performed, how much the procedure costs, advantages and disadvantages of the procedure, and how effective it is. Are there any barriers that might get in the way of people choosing this procedure? After gathering your information, create an informative pamphlet or brochure with this information. Present your final product to the class.
16. **Communicate with Others.** As a class, contact a person you know, in-person or online, who had a baby early in life (preferably before or during college). Think of several questions you would like answered and then interview this person about the experience. After the interview, write an essay describing what you learned.
17. **Make Decisions.** A crucial step in accomplishing your goals is getting the right support. To get this support, choose one trustworthy adult with whom you can have open conversations, even about sensitive topics. Once you have chosen this adult, write a brief statement addressed to the adult and explain your choice. In this statement, be sure to include your short- and long-terms goals and the topics you plan to discuss openly and honestly.

Describe what support you need from the adult and ask if the adult is comfortable with this role in your life. If you both agree, sign the statement. Keep it in a safe place so you can use it as a conversation starter when difficult topics arise.

18. **Set Goals.** Create a time line for your life. What are your goals for the next five years? the next 10 years? Do you want children? Remember that to reach your goals, you also need to set restrictions that will defend your goals and help you achieve them. Identify events or pressures that might deter you from living the life you have planned. Include events related to sexual activity and pregnancy. Then describe how you might avoid these obstacles.

19. **Practice Health-Enhancing Behaviors.** Knowing about contraception can not only protect your health, but can also help you promote the health of others. For each scenario given, write exactly what advice you would give to the friend asking you. Use what you learned in this chapter to help.

    A. Your friend, who is not dating anyone, is approached by an acquaintance at an event. This acquaintance clearly likes your friend and suggests going somewhere alone. Your friend asks to talk to you for a minute. What advice do you give?
    B. Two of your friends have been in a relationship for a year. They are two years apart, and the older partner has been sexually active in the past. Each friend comes to you separately looking for advice, since the couple is disagreeing about whether to be sexually active. What advice do you give each friend?

20. **Advocate for Health.** Create a social media campaign to outline the potential outcomes of unprotected sexual activity during the teen years. In your campaign, be sure to include risks related to pregnancy and STI transmission. Explain why sexual abstinence is a positive choice and also compare options for avoiding STI transmission and pregnancy.

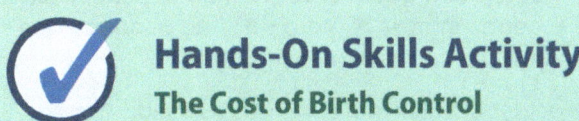

Hands-On Skills Activity
The Cost of Birth Control

Contraception can seem expensive to those who are buying it often or considering buying it. The costs of purchasing contraception are minimal, however, compared to the costs of giving birth to and caring for a baby or treating an incurable STI. In this activity, you will do research or visit local stores to compare the costs of purchasing contraception for one year versus the cost of having and caring for a baby for one year.

Steps for This Activity

1. Choose two contraceptive products discussed in this chapter. The products you choose should be available at a store or pharmacy. Research or estimate how often a person might need to purchase these products if the person was sexually active.

2. **Access Information.** Develop a comprehensive list that includes all the products a person would need to purchase to care for a newborn baby. Include cribs, carriers, baby clothes, and repeat purchases such as diapers, wipes, and food. Calculate the costs of the items on your list. Check prices online or go to local stores. Also research and record the cost of giving birth to a baby at your local hospital and getting testing and treatment for an incurable STI.

3. Multiply the cost of the contraceptive products you chose by the number of times a person would purchase them in one year of being sexually active. This is the cost of using contraception for one year. Then, add up the prices of the items a person would need to care for a newborn baby for one year. Make sure to multiply the costs of repeat purchases, such as diapers. Finally, add the cost of giving birth to a baby. Separately, add up the costs of testing and treatment for an incurable STI.

4. Compare the three total costs. How big is the difference between the cost of using contraception for one year and the cost of having and caring for a baby or getting testing and treatment for an STI? On a poster, write these numbers and attach pictures of all the items a person would purchase in each situation. Present your poster to the class.

Glossary/Glosario

English

B

barrier methods: contraceptive methods that prevent sperm from traveling through the female reproductive system and fertilizing an egg.

birth control implant: flexible, toothpick-sized contraceptive device inserted under the skin of the upper arm; releases progestin to stop ovulation.

birth control patch: plastic contraceptive device applied to the skin as a patch; releases hormones to stop ovulation.

birth control shot: contraceptive method in which a female receives an injection of progestin every three months to stop ovulation.

C

cervical cap: cup-shaped contraceptive device made of silicone; covers the cervix to prevent sperm from entering the uterus and is smaller than the diaphragm.

cisgender: identifying with the gender associated with one's biological sex.

contraception: any method that reduces the risk of pregnancy resulting from sexual activity.

contraceptive sponge: contraceptive device made of plastic foam; covers the cervix to prevent sperm from entering the uterus and contains spermicide.

D

diaphragm: cup-shaped contraceptive device made of silicone; covers the cervix to prevent sperm from entering the uterus and is bigger than the cervical cap.

disorder of sex development (DSD): condition of being born with or developing an ambiguous biological sex; also called a *difference of sex development (DSD)* or *intersex*.

Español

métodos de barrera: métodos anticonceptivos que evitan que los espermatozoides viajen a través del sistema reproductor femenino y fertilicen un óvulo.

implante anticonceptivo: dispositivo anticonceptivo flexible del tamaño de un mondadientes que se inserta debajo de la piel en la parte superior del brazo; libera progestina para detener la ovulación.

parche anticonceptivo: dispositivo anticonceptivo de plástico aplicado a la piel como parche; libera hormonas para detener la ovulación.

vacuna anticonceptiva: método anticonceptivo en el que la hembra recibe una inyección de progestina cada tres meses para detener la ovulación.

capuchón cervical: dispositivo anticonceptivo en forma de copa de silicona; cubre el cuello uterino para evitar que el esperma ingrese al útero y es más pequeño que el diafragma.

cisgénero: identificarse con el género asociado con el sexo biológico.

anticoncepción: cualquier método que reduzca el riesgo de embarazo como resultado de la actividad sexual.

esponja anticonceptiva: dispositivo anticonceptivo hecho de espuma plástica; cubre el cuello uterino para evitar que el esperma ingrese al útero y contiene espermicida.

diafragma: dispositivo anticonceptivo en forma de copa de silicona; cubre el cuello uterino para evitar que el esperma ingrese al útero y es más grande que el capuchón cervical.

trastorno del desarrollo sexual (disorder of sex development, DSD): condición de nacer o desarrollar un sexo biológico ambiguo; también se denomina *diferencia de desarrollo sexual (DSD)* o *intersexual*.

English

E

emergency contraception: contraceptive method used to prevent pregnancy when normal contraception has failed; includes the copper ParaGard® intrauterine device (IUD) and emergency contraceptive pills containing hormones.

F

fertility awareness method (FAM): contraceptive method that tracks a female's cycle of fertility and avoids sexual activity on days an egg can be fertilized.

G

gender binary: view that the genders of man and woman are entirely opposite; ignores gender expressions that fall between these opposites.

gender identity: component of identity that describes internal, deeply held thoughts and feelings about one's gender.

gender nonconforming: identifying with a gender that is not associated with one's biological sex.

H

homophobia: hostility, anger, exclusion, and violence directed at people who are LGBT+.

hormonal methods: contraceptive methods that alter a person's hormone levels to thicken cervical mucus and inhibit ovulation (the release of an egg).

human sexual response cycle: physical changes that occur in the body in response to sexual arousal and activity.

I

intrauterine device (IUD): small, T-shaped contraceptive device inserted into the uterus; copper IUDs interfere with sperm movement, and hormonal IUDs release hormones to thicken cervical mucus and inhibit ovulation.

Español

anticoncepción de emergencia: método anticonceptivo utilizado para prevenir el embarazo cuando la anticoncepción normal ha fallado; incluye el dispositivo intrauterino (DIU) ParaGard® de cobre y las píldoras anticonceptivas de emergencia que contienen hormonas.

método de conciencia de fertilidad (fertility awareness method, FAM): método anticonceptivo que controla el ciclo de fertilidad femenino y evita la actividad sexual en los días en que un óvulo puede ser fertilizado.

binarismo de género: razón que los géneros de hombre y mujer son completamente opuestos; ignora las expresiones de género que se encuentran entre estos opuestos.

identidad de género: componente de identidad que describe pensamientos y sentimientos internos y muy arraigados sobre su propio género.

no conformidad de género: identificarse con un género que no está asociado con el sexo biológico de uno.

homofobia: hostilidad, ira, exclusión y violencia dirigida a personas que están LGBT+.

métodos hormonales: métodos anticonceptivos que alteran los niveles hormonales de una persona para ensanchar mucosidad cervical y inhibir la ovulación (la liberación de un óvulo).

ciclo de respuesta sexual humana: cambios físicos que ocurren en el cuerpo en respuesta a la excitación y actividad sexual.

dispositivo intrauterino (DIU): pequeño dispositivo anticonceptivo en forma de T que se inserta en el útero; los DIU de cobre interfieren con el movimiento de los espermatozoides y los DIU hormonales liberan hormonas para ensanchar mucosidad cervical y inhibir la ovulación.

English

L

LGBT+: acronym used to identify people who are nonheterosexual and/or gender nonconforming.

M

masturbation: self-stimulation of the reproductive organs in response to sexual excitement.

N

natural methods: contraceptive methods that time sexual activity with a female's menstrual cycle and the sexual response cycle to prevent the sperm and egg from meeting.

nonbinary: identifying with a gender that falls outside the categories of man or woman.

O

oral contraceptives: medications containing hormones that stop ovulation; are taken every day.

orgasm: climax of sexual excitement characterized by pleasurable muscular contractions in the reproductive organs and throughout the body.

S

same-sex marriage: legal marriage between two people of the same biological sex.

sexual history: information about a person's past sexual activity and partners.

sexuality: element of identity that includes a person's biological sex, gender identity and expression, sexual orientation, and sexual experiences and thoughts.

sexual orientation: enduring pattern of a person's romantic and/or sexual attraction to other people.

spermicide: substance that inactivates sperm.

sterilization: contraceptive method that permanently prevents pregnancy by altering the reproductive system, often through surgery.

Español

LGBT+: acrónimo utilizado para identificar personas no heterosexuales y/o sin conformidad de género.

masturbación: autoestimulación de los órganos reproductivos como respuesta a la excitación sexual.

métodos naturales: métodos anticonceptivos que regulan la actividad sexual en función del ciclo menstrual femenino y el ciclo de respuesta sexual para evitar que el esperma y el óvulo se encuentren.

no binario: identificarse con un género que queda fuera de las categorías de hombre o mujer.

anticonceptivos orales: medicamentos que contienen hormonas que detienen la ovulación; se toman todos los días.

orgasmo: clímax de excitación sexual caracterizado por contracciones musculares placenteras en los órganos reproductivos y en todo el cuerpo.

matrimonio del mismo sexo: matrimonio legal entre dos personas del mismo sexo biológico.

historia sexual: información sobre la actividad sexual pasada de una persona y sus parejas.

sexualidad: elemento de identidad que incluye el sexo biológico, identidad y expresión de género, orientación sexual y experiencias y pensamientos sexuales de una persona.

orientación sexual: patrón duradero de la atracción romántica y/o sexual de una persona hacia otras personas.

espermicida: sustancia que inactiva el esperma.

esterilización: método anticonceptivo que previene de forma permanente el embarazo al alterar el sistema reproductivo, a menudo mediante cirugía.

English

T

transgender: identifying with the gender opposite the one that is associated with one's biological sex.

tubal ligation: surgical procedure that cuts or blocks the fallopian tubes, permanently preventing pregnancy.

V

vaginal ring: flexible, ring-shaped contraceptive device inserted into the vagina; releases hormones to stop ovulation.

vasectomy: surgical procedure that cuts or blocks the vas deferens, permanently preventing pregnancy.

W

withdrawal: contraceptive method that involves pulling the penis out of the vagina before ejaculation.

Español

transgénero: identificarse con el género opuesto al que está asociado con el sexo biológico de uno.

ligadura de trompas: procedimiento quirúrgico que corta o bloquea las trompas de Falopio, evitando permanentemente el embarazo.

anillo vaginal: dispositivo anticonceptivo flexible con forma de anillo insertado en la vagina; libera hormonas para detener la ovulación.

vasectomía: procedimiento quirúrgico que corta o bloquea los conductos deferentes, evitando permanentemente el embarazo.

abstinencia/retiro: método anticonceptivo que consiste en sacar el pene de la vagina antes de la eyaculación.

Index

A
agender, 805
androgynous, 805
androromantic, 806
androsexual, 806
aromantic, 806
asexual, 806

B
basal body temperature, 847–848
bias, 809, 828
bigender, 805
biological sex, 803–804
biromantic, 806
birth control. *See* contraception
birth control implant, 840, 843
birth control patch, 840, 842
birth control pill. *See* oral contraceptives
birth control shot, 840, 843
bisexual, 806
Byrd, James, Jr., 809

C
Centers for Disease Control and Prevention (CDC), 831
cervical cap, 834, 838
cervical mucus, 848
cervix, 837–838
cisgender, 805
Civil Rights Act of 1991, 809
Civil Service Reform Act of 1978, 809
closeted, 807
combination pill, 841–842
"coming out," 808
condoms, 835–836
continuous birth control, 841–842
contraception
    birth control implant, 840, 843
    birth control patch, 840, 842
    birth control shot, 840, 843
    cervical cap, 834, 838
    contraceptive sponge, 834, 837
    diaphragm, 834, 837–838
    emergency, 840, 844–845
    external condoms, 834–836
    fertility awareness methods (FAM), 847–848
    internal condoms, 834, 836
    intrauterine device (IUD), 840, 843
    oral contraceptives, 840–842
    reliable information about, 828f
    selecting, 830–832
    sexual abstinence, 818, 830, 832
    spermicide, 834–835
    sterilization, 830, 847, 849–851
    vaginal ring, 840, 842
    withdrawal, 847, 849
contraceptive sponge, 834, 837
culture, 814

D
decision-making, 817–818
demiromantic, 806
demisexual, 806
diaphragm, contraception, 834, 837–838
difference of sex development. *See* disorder of sex development
discrimination, 807–808
disorder of sex development (DSD), 803
diversity, 804–810
DSD (disorder of sex development), 803

E
ejaculation, 813
emergency contraception, 830, 840, 844–845
erection, 813
estrogen, 839
extended-cycle birth control, 841–842
external condoms, 834–836

F
fallopian tubes, 850
family relationships, 814
FAM (fertility awareness methods), 847–848
female sterilization, 847, 850–851
femininity, 804–805
fertility awareness methods (FAM), 847–848

G
gay. *See* LGBT+
gay straight alliance (GSA), 808
gender, 804–805
gender binary, 804–805
gender expression, 805
gender fluid, 805
gender identity, 805, 807–810

Note: Page numbers followed by *f* indicate figures.

gender neutral, 805
gender nonconforming, 805
gender queer, 805
gender questioning, 805
gender roles, 804
gender stereotypes, 802, 804
goals and goal setting, 815
GSA (gay straight alliance), 808
gyneromantic, 806
gynesexual, 806

H

hate crimes, 809
health information, 828f, 831
heteroromantic, 806
heterosexual, 806
homophobia, 808
homoromantic, 806
homosexual, 806
hormones, 839
human sexual response cycle, 812–813

I

influences on sexual behavior, 813–816
internal condoms, 834, 836
intrauterine devices (IUDs), 840, 843
IUDs (intrauterine devices), 843

K

Klinefelter Syndrome, 803

L

latex allergy, 835
laws
    anti-discrimination, 809
    Civil Rights Act of 1991, 809
    Civil Service Reform Act of 1978, 809
    Matthew Shepard and James Byrd, Jr., Hate Crimes Prevention Act, 809
lesbian. *See* LGBT+
LGBT+
    discrimination against, 807–808
    hate crimes, 809
    laws protecting individuals, 809
    safe-zone programs, 810
    support for, 808–810
lubricants, 835

M

male sterilization, 847, 850
marriage, 809
masculinity, 804–805

masturbation, 812
Matthew Shepard and James Byrd, Jr., Hate Crimes Prevention Act, 809
media, 814–816, 827, 829
minipill. *See* progestin-only pill
myths and facts, 828–829

N

nocturnal emissions, 812
nonbinary, 805
norms, 814

O

oral contraceptives, 840–842, 844
orgasm, 813
ovaries, 865
ovulation, 839–844, 847–848
oxytocin, 816, 818

P

panromantic, 806
pansexual, 806
peer pressure, 814
penis, 813, 835, 849
polyromantic, 806
polysexual, 806
pre-ejaculate fluid, 849
pregnancy prevention. *See* contraception; sexual abstinence
prejudice, 807–808
progestin, 839
progestin-only pill, 842
protective factors, 813–815
puberty, 812

Q

questioning, sexual orientation, 807

R

relationships
    influence on health, 814
        making decisions in, 818–819
reliable sources of health information, 828f, 831
reproductive health. *See* sexual health
risk factors, 813–815
romantic attraction, 806
romantic orientation, 806

S

safe zones, 810
same-sex marriage, 809
same-sex parents, 809
semen, 835–836

sexual abstinence
    benefits of, 818, 830, 832
    challenges to, 832
    practicing, 818
sexual activity
    benefits of abstinence, 818, 830, 832
    consequences of, 815–816
    decision-making about, 817–818
    discussing with a partner, 818
    factors affecting, 813–815
    preventing pregnancy, 826–851
sexual assault, 844
sexual attraction, 806
sexual health
    abstinence, 818, 830, 832
    answering questions about, 831
    contraception, 826–851
sexual history, 818
sexual intercourse. *See* sexual activity
sexuality
    biological sex, 803–804
    gender identity, 804–805
    sexual activity, 813–819
    sexual feelings, 811–812
    sexual orientation, 806–807
sexually transmitted diseases (STDs). *See* sexually transmitted infections (STIs)
sexually transmitted infections (STIs), 830, 832, 835–836
sexual maturity. *See* puberty
sexual orientation, 806–807
sexual relationships
    consequences of, 815–818
    making decisions in, 818–819

sexual response cycle, 812–813
Shepard, Matthew, 809
skolioromantic, 806
skoliosexual, 806
spermicide, 834–835
stereotypes, 802, 804
sterilization, 830, 847, 849–851
STDs (sexually transmitted diseases). *See* STIs (sexually transmitted infections)
STIs (sexually transmitted infections), 830, 832, 835–836

T

transgender, 805
tubal ligation, 847, 850–851
Turner Syndrome, 803

U

upstanders, 808
uterus, 843

V

vagina, 813, 836–838, 842
vaginal ring, 840, 842
values, 815
vas deferens, 850
vasectomy, 847, 850

W

wet dreams, 812
withdrawal bleeding, 842
withdrawal, contraception, 847, 849